CHILDBIRTH EDUCATION:
A Nursing Perspective

CHILDBIRTH EDUCATION:
A Nursing Perspective

JEANNETTE L. SASMOR, R.N., Ed.D., F.A.A.N.
Certified Childbirth Educator
Founder of the American Society
of Childbirth Educators

A WILEY MEDICAL PUBLICATION
JOHN WILEY & SONS
New York / Chichester / Brisbane / Toronto

Library of Congress Cataloging in Publication Data:

Sasmor, Jeannette L.
    Childbirth education.

    1.   Childbirth—Study and teaching.
    2.   Obstetrical nursing.   I.   Title.
    [DNLM: 1.   Obstetrics—Education—Nursing texts.
    2.   Labor—Nursing texts.   3.   Parents—Education—
    Nursing texts.   WY18.3 S252c]

    RG973.S37   610.73′678   78-32117
    ISBN 0-471-75490-0

Printed in the United States of America

10 9 8 7 6 5 4 3 2 1

This book is dedicated to the idea that family-centered obstetrical care is a right that the consumer can expect.

Although not all consumers want family-centered care, all those who seek it should find it as a regular condition of modern obstetrical care.

Contributors

ROSEMARY COLUMBO, R.N., B.S.
Assistant Director of Staff
Development and Childbirth Educator
St. Anthony's Hospital
St. Petersburg, Florida

JANET GAUVAIN, R.N., B.S.
Director, Adolescent Education Program
Maternity Department
Sarasota County Health Department
Sarasota, Florida

JONNA JUNG, R.N., B.S.
Member, Child Development Center
and Adolescent Education Program
Maternity Department
Sarasota County Health Department
Sarasota, Florida

PAMELA LAMPERELLI, M.S.W.
Social Worker, Maurawood Residence
West Palm Beach, Florida

JAMES C. SASMOR, B.S.
Corporate Secretary
The American Society of Childbirth Educators
Tampa, Florida

JANE M. SMITH, R.N., C.C.E.
Counselor and Childbirth Educator
Maurawood Residence
West Palm Beach, Florida

MARGARET Z. TAYLOR, R.N., M.N.Ed.
Formerly Assistant Professor for Parent-Child Nursing
College of Nursing
University of South Florida
Tampa, Florida

THOMAS J. VALIN, M.D.
Obstetrician in Private Practice and Medical Advisor
Childbirth Education Association
of the Palm Beaches
West Palm Beach, Florida

Foreword

Jeannette Sasmor, Ed.D., the author of this book, was first introduced to me a few years ago by a mutual friend, Dr. Howard Jacobsen, a professor of obstetrics at Harvard University. At that time she was working to raise the level of consciousness of nurses and physicians about childbirth education and to increase their participation in this growing area of consumer interest. Since that first meeting, much growth has taken place, both in members and sophistication, in the prepared childbirth education movement. No small amount of credit must go to Dr. Sasmor, whose book provides a clearly marked route to enable all nurses involved in the care of mothers and infants to participate in this movement.

Dr. Sasmor carries the reader through the development of the childbirth education movement in the United States from its inception through 1978. Different schools of thought are treated lucidly without making value judgments. A knowledge of the different techniques and philosophies of childbirth education enables the nurse to support the parents' efforts, whichever approach to psychoprophylaxis they follow. This flexibility is particularly important for the nurse working in labor and delivery who often has not had prior contact with the client. The nurse working in intrapartal care often has her initial introduction to the family after labor has begun and when the family is in stress.

The chapter on planning for childbirth education programs will provide an excellent review for the educator and guide for the novice to the educational process. Steps in planning, implementing, and evaluating are thoughtfully developed, reinforcing a process model.

The unit on support systems brings the reader back from the conceptual framework to the realities of client care. Thomas Valin, M.D., discusses needs and approaches to resolution that should be read by all nurses and physicians. The direct and indirect approaches he suggests for facilitating change are handled in a forthright manner.

Jim Sasmor's description of needs and feelings of the participating expectant father should acquaint all health professionals with the father's need for support and reassurance. He makes the point that the attitudes and conduct of the nurse are powerful influences in the performance of the father. One might carry this thought one step further and submit for the reader's consideration that the conduct of the father has an important effect on the performance of the mother. The chapter on the single mother provides some helpful hints to caregivers, and the needs of the parents of a high-risk infant are sensitively handled. The book concludes with a section on patterns of development and options for the profession in the future.

This is a book for nurses about nursing. It is timely in its approach in reflecting the changing structure of the American family. Dr. Sasmor's book is based on sound principles of education. The message is clear without being judgmental. It provides an organized approach to the integration of the nursing process with the process of childbirth education. This book can be highly recommended for nurses in practice as well as for students interested in improving maternal-infant care.

Mitzi L. Duxbury, R.N., Ph.D., F.A.A.N.
Associate Professor
Assistant Dean for Graduate Studies
University of Minnesota School of Nursing

Preface

The intent of this book is to place childbirth education within its proper perspective, the practice of nursing. As an active member of the childbirth education movements in the United States since the mid-1960s, I have been aware of an artificial dichotomy created between the grass roots demands for more meaningful childbirth education and the institutional practices influencing the delivery of services. Historically, nurses have provided the bulk of childbirth education through hospitals or community agencies. Although other professionals and lay persons have attempted to provide aspects of childbirth education, the major role is still played by nurses. This book, I believe, explains the integral relationship between the educational process that is childbirth education and the nursing process itself, with its strong emphasis on health promotion and health maintenance.

This is a book written for nurses about nursing. It is an application of the basic theory of nursing to the specific practice of the nurse who is a childbirth educator. Intended for any nurse entering the field of childbirth education, this book explains how the field developed and how the practice falls within the parameters of nursing. It examines the interactive process of education as well as the interpersonal responsibilities between practitioner and client and between practitioner and the other professionals assisting the client.

This book is not a cookbook. It offers no single recipe to meet all educational needs. It provides a theoretical framework for professional practice. One hallmark of the professional is the ability to make knowledgable decisions. It is the purpose of this book to assist the professional nurse in making knowledgable decisions about the practice of childbirth education.

Jeannette L. Sasmor, R.N., Ed.D., F.A.A.N.
Certified Childbirth Educator

Prologue

Culture is perpetually on a road in time. The path behind represents traditional roles and modes of doing things; the path ahead represents emerging roles and new modes of behavior. Some of us will never be able to leave the path behind us to move ahead. Some of us will go forward now and will assume the traditional role of a future time. And some of us will go forward now and continue to choose the emerging role each time we arrive at a decisive point in time.

Nursing culture has survived several decision points in the recent past. Emerging roles in the practice of nursing are appearing in every area of interest. As a service profession, nursing has had to respond to both the vastly increasing body of technological knowledge and the changing demands of the public being served. So it is in maternity care. Technology has increased the potential for physical safety of mother and baby. With survival no longer the only concern, public interest has also shifted focus. Ever-increasing numbers of expectant parents are seeking satisfying as well as safe experiences in the birth of their children. Traditional nursing has provided direct care that emphasized physical safety through diet counseling and implementation of the medical management program. But in order for current public demands to be satisfied, the emerging role for nursing in this area will need to encompass more. Society has changed. Parents have changed. Nursing must respond to the changes in constructive ways that consider both parental desires and the existing parameters of safe maternity care. If nurses do not respond quickly enough or in large enough numbers to meet the needs of parents, parents will find other sources for satisfying these needs.

Childbirth education has long been a part of nursing care to parents during the maternity cycle. Whether it continues to remain a specialty area of nursing practice will depend on the responsiveness of the professional practitioner. As in every area of professional practice, childbirth education should represent the sound application of scientifically based theoretical knowledge to specific situations.

This is a point in time when nursing has the option of clinging to traditional roles or moving ahead and accepting emerging roles, roles that will demand high-level professional practice. As a childbirth educator, a nurse is not only a disseminator of information but also a catalyst whose primary role is to ease the transition that expectant parents make when they assume the responsibilities of parenthood.

Contents

CHILDBIRTH EDUCATION:
A Nursing Perspective

PART ONE

WHAT IS CHILDBIRTH EDUCATION?

Part I provides a broad foundation for understanding childbirth education that serves as a basis for the subsequent chapters. Just as an individual is a product of biological, psychological and sociological drives that interrelate to create the whole, so the childbirth education movement is a product of the forces of historical and social change. Chapter 1 deals with these forces and how they have contributed to the current state of the art.

The focus of Chapter 2 is the theoretical basis on which the practice of childbirth education rests. As with its evolution, the theoretical basis of childbirth education also stems from several sources. Adult learning theory, stress-adaption theory, and crisis intervention theory each contribute a valuable facet to making a viable theoretical framework that explains childbirth education.

The final chapter in this part, Chapter 3, is a practical review of the three major approaches extant in childbirth education today: Read, Lamaze, and Eclectic. Rather than an attempt to endorse any one approach, this chapter presents all three so that a nurse relating to prepared parents either antepartally in a maternity clinic or physician's office, or intrapartally during the labor process, can knowledgeably answer questions and offer support to the approach that the parents have chosen.

The information in this part is designed to provide any nurse seeking knowledge about childbirth education with a broad overview of the historical development of the field in the United States, an intellectual appreciation of the theoretical support for childbirth education, and a working knowledge of the main approaches to preparation for labor and delivery.

Chapter 1

Societal Changes

The childbearing process is an expected part of life in the human species. Over the centuries of recorded history, the process has been invested with magical properties that have reflected the level of technological development of the particular era in question. In today's world, it is no different. Childbirth is surrounded by magical rites and rituals that modern society has assigned to the temple of the medicine man—the modern hospital.[1,2] Thus, even at our level of civilization the normalcy of the process is lost.

Despite the human tendency to preserve the mystical protection against the unknown, there is an ever-increasing group of parents who do not wish to lose either normal perspective of childbirth or their identity as thinking adults, which is frequently sacrificed on the medical altar. These groups of parents, who belong to no single geographic location, are a product of advancing history and social change.

EMERGING ROLES

During the past generation, changing roles have been developing for the expanding family and its members. Many expectant and new parents are no

1. Doris Haire, *The Cultural Warping of Childbirth* (Milwaukee: International Childbirth Education Association, 1972).
2. N. S. Shaw, *Forced Labor: Maternity Care in the United States* (New York: Pergamon Press, 1974).

3

longer following the traditional roles that their own parents assumed, either in the care of the child in the family or in the actual process of childbearing.[3] Unisex and the de-emphasis of sex roles have permitted men to assume more active roles in the family, particularly during and after the birth of a child.

The emerging roles for the members of the expanding family emphasize knowledgeable participation of both mother and father during the labor process for mutual support. This role for the mother as parturient using self-help tools can be more readily accepted as an extension of the traditionally more passive role. The emerging role of the father as labor coach represents a greater breach with the traditional role of the expectant, which was an extension of the traditional role of the man in American society and virtually excluded his participation in a female rite of passage—childbirth.

Since the beginning of this century the family as a unit of societal organization has changed in America. An identifiable shift has emerged from the traditional institution-type of family to one that serves as a person-centered unit providing companionship. This changing pattern has led to a shift from a family of father-centered control to what has been described as a family of shared control and decision-making. This phenomenon is found to a greater extent among families in the middle and upper economic classes of American society, although it is found to a lesser degree in those families of lower socioeconomic status in which the men are participating more in what were traditionally female roles in the home.[4]

These shifts within the family role structure have occurred at the same time as the intergenerational relationships have weakened. The increased tempo of living in a superindustrialized society combined with nomadic conditions of geographic mobility have taken their toll on the relationships that can be built by family members.[5] As a result, the new American family has become the most isolated, while at the same time the most dependent, of any family type in the history of this nation. In effect, the nuclear family has been enucleated. The isolation from the resources of the traditional family model leads parents to seek help from professionals, from literature, and from each other instead of depending on what had been done in the past as a part of their family tradition or instead of seeking advice from their own parents, grandparents, aunts, or other older relations.[6]

The expanding family today, therefore, places greater stress on outside sources such as formalized childbirth education, and the formalized childbirth education programs are also a product of sociological evolution. Childbirth

3. Angela B. McBride, "Can the Family Survive?" *American Journal of Nursing* (October, 1975).
4. Lee Rainwater, *Family Design* (Chicago: Aldine, 1965), p. 278.
5. Alvin Tofler, *Future Shock* (New York: Random House, 1970).
6. E. E. LeMasters, *Parents in Modern America* (Homewood Ill: The Dorsey Press, 1970).

education itself is very much subject to the social forces created by changing times. Social patterns are woven into the history that forms the basis for action in the present world. Examination of the past can often help to make the present more comprehensible.

CHILDBIRTH EDUCATION HISTORY

The historical precedent for formalized childbirth education is linked in time with the development of obstetrics as an identifiable medical specialty practice. From time immemorial, the business of having babies and rearing children was considered part of a woman's lot in life, and her mother and other female relatives were expected to pass on these female mysteries to her. Woman-to-woman childbirth education was a sharing of experiences, good or bad, usually representing a process of mutual ignorance highlighted with some truths, many half-truths, and a myriad of old wives' tales that helped to make the unknown less fearful. This kind of behavior was, of course, completely appropriate to times in which female sexuality was considered scandalous and accurate knowledge of the functionings of the human body was severely limited.

As times changed, the social clime began to change. Women were accorded enough status to be considered worthy of education and able to benefit from it. At the same time, the social configurations in America shifted from rural agricultural to urban industrial with the result that large multigenerational families gave way to the more isolated single-generation families of procreation. This structural change left the young wife with a limited support system, if any was present at all.

Red Cross Program

The first organization to realize that an educational gap existed and to act on it was the American National Red Cross.[7] In 1908 the Red Cross in Washington, D.C. began a course in home health and hygiene nursing, the fifth part of which was concerned with mother and baby. These first formal classes in

7.   Jeannette L. Sasmor, "The Future of Childbirth Education," presented to the First National Convention of the Nurses Association of the American College of Obstetricians and Gynecologists, Las Vegas, Nevada, 1974.

childbirth education included the care of the expectant and new mother, and the care of the new baby and diet. The course of study met with such success that the program was promoted nationally in 1913. By 1919 the Red Cross had expanded this program by preparing nursing aids for a public health nursing program that promoted individual parent education. It was this very program that was the forerunner of the Public Health Service. It was also this program that served as the precedent for childbirth education as a community-based service, because, at the time of the Red Cross program, hospitalization for confinement was unheard of.

Maternity Center Association

The Great Depression wreaked havoc on the status quo of Americans. One of the positive outcomes was the realization that some male and female roles were interchangeable. Jobs were scarce. It was not uncommon for a woman to work and her husband to be unemployed. As a result of this social and economic phenomenon, some men began to re-examine their traditional roles. When, in 1938, the Maternity Center Association opened classes for expectant parents, many couples came.[8] Word of mouth has kept these classes in demand ever since.

"Natural Childbirth" Movement

Following World War II, hospitalization for childbearing became more generally accepted. Medical advances, both pharmacological and operative, could offer the mother greater comfort and the infant greater assurance of survival. During this postwar period grass roots movement developed and began to build momentum. This movement was probably a response to the implications of "interfering with nature" surrounding hospitalization for labor and delivery. "Natural Childbirth" became a goal for an increasing number of women around the world. The work of Dr. Grantly Dick-Read became known and gained in popularity among women.[9] In teaching his concept of childbirth without fear, Dick-Read's goal was to emphasize the naturalness of the birth experience and to promote the idea that having a baby can be a happy, healthy experience. This educational approach was a primary step in moving toward participatory roles for parents in the childbirth experience. It is only in accepting the idea that the pregnant woman is not sick despite her need for medical management that one can then accept family-centered maternity

8.   Martin Kelly, "Schools for Parenthood," *Expecting* (Fall, 1972), p. 16.
9.   Grantly Dick-Read, *Childbirth Without Fear*, 2nd ed. (New York: Harper & Row, 1959).

care not as an aberration of traditional obstetrical practice but as a normal, natural part of the life cycle of a family unit.

In the years that followed, women who had had what they considered "successful" experiences banded together, some with the assistance of knowledgeable professionals, some without any support, to offer information and training to other women. These groups for childbirth education eventually consolidated into a federation of groups known as the International Childbirth Education Association, which serves as a core for a variety of philosophies and approaches represented in its constituent member groups.

The Psychoprophylactic Method of Education for Childbirth

About the time I.C.E.A. was coming into its own, another school of thinking appeared. Disenchanted with the claims and subsequent "failures" of the Read method, disciples of the French doctor, Fernand Lamaze, introduced the psychoprophylactic, or childbirth-without-pain, or Lamaze, method to America.[10] The formation of the American Society for Psychoprophylaxis in Obstetrics in New York and the Childbirth Without Pain Education Association in Detroit represented two approaches to psychoprophylaxis, related and yet different. But, the importance of their appearance and growth lies in the interest of parents in participating in the birth experience, not merely allowing nature to take its course, but actually taking an active role in assisting nature with as little artificial intervention as is safe and necessary. As in prior generations, this kind of behavior is appropriate to the times in which these parents live.

RESPONSES TO CHILDBIRTH EDUCATION

However, parents alone, no matter how strong their interest, will never be able to revolutionize the practice of obstetrics. They need help from the inside of the professions. Throughout its period of development, childbirth education has remained a service primarily outside of the hospital structure. A grass roots movement gone wild, childbirth education as a means of promoting family-centered maternity care was a need increasingly expressed by parents over the past 20 years. It was the unresponsiveness of the professional

10. Marjorie Karmel, *Thank You, Dr. Lamaze* (New York: Dolphin, 1965).

establishment that forced parents to seek relief through the law. The most startling development was a bill introduced and reintroduced into the House of Representatives in Congress, which, if passed into law, would make it mandatory for all hospitals receiving Federal funds to permit the father in labor and delivery with the permission of the mother and physician.[11] This situation is fraught with conflict born of a desire to change an unresponsive system by dictum.

Changing a system from the outside rarely meets with lasting success.[12] In an attempt to improve communication and understanding among professionals about childbirth education, the American Society of Childbirth Educators was formed in 1971. This organization was the first professional association for childbirth education as a family experience. Unlike other public service organizations already existing in this field, the A.S.C.E. had as its primary goal to serve the professional caring for expectant and new parents. A collaborative organization, it offered membership to physicians and registered nurses who share this special interest in the hopes of achieving a better understanding of parent goals by bringing together the professionals dealing with expectant and new parents. Through understanding and acceptance, rather than unsuccessful demands from outside, perhaps change in the health care delivery serving this segment of the population will emerge. For this to occur it will be necessary to overcome one of the external obstacles created by well-meaning people whose lack of understanding has led to the present situation.

THE CHILDBIRTH TEAM CONCEPT

The concept of the childbirth team is one that has been incorporated into a variety of preparations for labor classes. However, because childbirth education has so often existed outside the setting where the childbirth experience occurs, the team concept has not always been accurate nor always accepted by all members of the team. Further, the original team concept was a "troika," made up of three components—the doctor, the teacher, and the parents (Fig. 1–1).[13] This distortion of role theory has omitted one essential member of the childbirth team—the labor nurse—and it has lumped together two other members whose roles and functions are distinctly different—the prepared mother and the prepared father (Fig. 1–2). Is it any wonder that

11.   H. R. Bill 1502, Congress of the United States, January 9, 1973.
12.   Alvin Zander, "Resistance to Change—Its Analysis and Prevention," in *Changing Organizational Behavior*, Alton C. Bartlett and Thomas A. Kayser, eds., (Englewood Cliffs, N.J.: Prentice-Hall, 1973).
13.   Heinz L. Luchinski, "Psychoprophylaxis: Involvement Encouraged," *Ob-Gyn Observer* (July, 1970), p. 2.

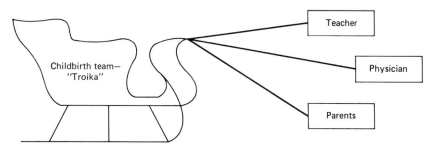

Figure 1–1.

The Childbirth Team—a Troika Concept.

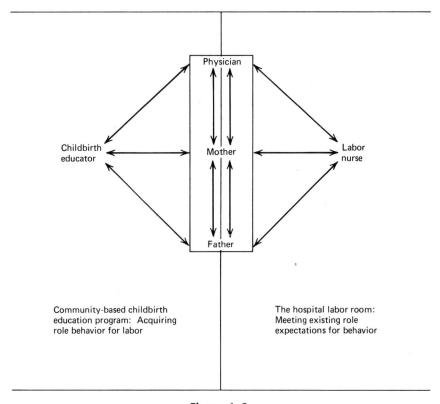

Figure 1–2.

In the developing childbirth education movement, the communication breakdown existed because the childbirth educator and the labor nurse did not interact.

parents who have been taught to behave as a prepared woman and as a labor coach by one person feel tension and conflict when they are met by another person who expects them to behave as patient and visitor? This situation is further compounded by expectations that the parents may develop regarding resistance by the hospital personnel. Informed consent and parent power, while laudable goals, should not be the battle banners of parents whose main objective should be to support each other during the stresses of the birth of their child. All too often it is exactly this kind of situation that fosters a spirit of competition between parents and the medical team instead of the needed spirit of cooperation essential to the true goal of prepared childbirth—a healthy, happy experience.

SUMMARY

The trends of education for responsible parenthood point to dynamic response to parent needs. In the early days of childbirth education, the need was for general information about pregnancy and the newborn; this education gradually came to include fathers as well as mothers in the baby-care classes. The concept of family-centered care grew as interest spread to the specific means for coping with labor and delivery; the most recent development has been the expressed desire to learn about and develop parenting skills beyond the physical care of the newborn. Childbirth education has grown and developed in response to the needs of parents. Each development has served as a building block for the next so that professionally taught quality courses today offer parents learning experiences in all three domains of human experience—cognitive, affective, and psychomotor. Childbirth educators capable of offering quality experiences for parent growth must have teaching skills and knowledge of the teaching–learning process as it applies to adult learners as well as a considerable fund of information about the process of childbearing and the means for coping with it.

BIBLIOGRAPHY

——, "ASPO Convention," *Baby Talk*: August, 1977.

——, "Childbearing is a Family Affair," *American Baby Magazine:* June, 1972.

Arms S: *Immaculate Deception*. Boston, Houghton-Mifflin, 1975.

Bam SL: "Adrogyny vs the Tight Little Lives of Fluffy Women & Chesty Men," *Psychology Today* **9**:4, Sept, 1975.

Bean C: *Methods of Childbirth*. New York, Doubleday, 1972.

Bean C: *Labor & Delivery, An Observer's Diary.* New York, Doubleday, 1977.

Bing E, Colman L: *Making Love During Pregnancy.* New York, Bantam Books, 1978.

Boston Women's Health Book Collective: *Our Bodies, Ourselves.* New York, Simon & Schuster, 1973.

Devitt N: "The Transition from Home to Hospital Birth in the United States, 1930–1960," *Birth and The Family Journal* **4**:3, Summer, 1977.

Dock L, Stewart IM: *A Short History of Nursing from Its Earliest Times to Present Day.* New York, G. P. Putnam & Sons, 1920.

Elkins VH: *The Rights of Pregnant Parents.* New York, Two Continents, 1976.

Frank LK: *On the Importance of Infancy.* New York, Random House, 1966.

Goode WJ: *The Family.* Englewood Cliffs, NJ, Prentice-Hall, 1964.

Goodrich F: *Preparing for Childbirth.* Englewood Cliffs, NJ, Prentice-Hall, 1966.

Green G: *The Female Eunuch.* New York, McGraw-Hill, 1970.

Guttmacher, AF: *Pregnancy, Birth and Family Planning.* New York, Signet Books, 1973.

Haire J: "The Age of Consumerism in Maternity Care," ICEA News, Sept/Oct, 1970.

Heardman H: *A Way to Natural Childbirth.* Edinburgh, F & S Livingstone, 1970.

Hungerford MJ: *Childbirth Education,* Springfield, Ill, Charles C Thomas, 1972.

Jenning LG: "The Changing Health Care Needs of Women: Clinical Specialists Take Heed," *JOGN* **6**:3, May/Jun, 1977.

Kelly M: "School for Parenthood," *Expecting,* Fall, 1972.

Lang R: *Birth Book.* Ben Lomond, Calif: Genesis Press, 1972.

Langman L, et al: *Natural Childbirth as a Social Movement,* speech presented to the First Meeting of the Psychosomatic Ob-Gyn Society, Philadelphia, Pa., January, 1972.

Liley HMI, Day B: *Modern Motherhood.* New York, Random House, 1969.

McKilligan HR: *The First Day of Life.* New York, Springer Publishing Co., 1970.

Montague A: *Life Before Birth.* New York, Dell Publishing, 1966.

Mousseau J: "The Family Pursor of Love," *Psychology Today* **9**:3, August, 1975.

Nilsson L: *A Child Is Born: The Drama of Life Before Birth.* New York, Dell Publishing, 1966.

Otto SE: "ICEA: The Challenges of Childbirth Education. . . Yesterday, Today, Tomorrow," *Mother's Manual* **14**:1, Jan/Feb, 1978.

Rakowitz E: "ASPO: Birth & Growth of An Ideal," *Mother's Manual,* **14**:1, Jan/Feb, 1978.

Richardson SA, Guttmacher AF: eds., *Childbearing—Its Social and Psychological Aspects.* Baltimore, Williams & Wilkins, 1967.

Spock BM: *Problem of Parents.* New York, Crest Books, 1962.

Wertz RW, Wertz DC: *Lying in: A History of Childbirth in America.* New York, The Free Press, 1977.

Wuerger M: "The Young Adult: Stepping Into Parenthood," *Am J Nursing* **76**:8, August, 1976.

Chapter 2

A Theoretical Basis for Childbirth Education

The proliferation of childbirth education programs in the past decade has led to considerable confusion among both the public and professionals about the efficacy of any one approach. Each method often holds rigidly to its own principles, disclaiming the general applicability of any of the other approaches. This attitude has frequently added emotional overtones to the existing confusion in the minds of expectant parents seeking the "best" method. It has led professionals to doubt the validity of any approach to prepared childbirth and to provide limited support to parents who wholeheartedly endorse any particular approach.

This proliferation, however, was a direct response to public demand for adequate preparation for childbirth, as a result of which a variety of programs have sprouted throughout the country. European methods are directly applied in some educational programs and bear the names of the developers—Read, Lamaze, Wright.[1,2,3] Practitioners in other programs have steadfastly insisted that they do not follow one method and choose to call their courses "Preparation for Childbirth" and "Preparation for Labor and Delivery," but these are usually based on a modification of one or more of the European methods.

1. Grantly Dick-Read, *Childbirth Without Fear*, 2nd ed. (New York: Harper & Row, 1959).
2. Fernand Lamaze, *Painless Childbirth* (Chicago: Henry Regnery, 1970).
3. Erna Wright, *The New Childbirth* (New York: Hart Publishing Co., 1966).

UNIFYING CHILDBIRTH EDUCATION APPROACHES

In attempting to understand the essence of childbirth education, it is imperative to turn away momentarily from the CONTENT of childbirth education to the PROCESS of childbirth education, because it is in the process that the similarities of the various methods find common ground.

Leon Chertok, in his discourse on the various programs of psychophysiologic preparation for childbearing, stresses the value of preparing the expectant mother and fulfilling her particular needs.[4] Yet, even though he recognizes the similarities in the programs, Chertok fails to emphasize the consistent commonalities in all of the approaches to educated birth:

1. Factual information about human reproduction, detailed descriptions of the processes of labor and delivery.
2. Controlled relaxation, and
3. Specific learned breathing techniques to be used in response to the labor sensations.

These three commonalities are the basis for the theoretical interpretation to be discussed here. The theoretical framework for the discussion is the Stress Theory, which is based on an understanding of human behavior and the ability to cope with stress.[5,6,7] Viewing childbirth education as a means of stress adaptation is broadly applicable to each method because it explains the overall process of preparation for childbirth. Even though each approach claims a theory to rationalize its particular method, the method-specific approaches are usually inadequate to explain more than a part of an approach and often cannot explain the efficacy of other methods.

To establish a general theoretical base for understanding childbirth education, it was necessary to look at the general needs of the expectant mother during parturition. Crawford demonstrated that anxiety could interfere with the process of labor and should be alleviated.[8] Anxiety, after all, becomes a prolonged stressor on the body if not lessened. But is not labor a normal

4. Leon Chertok, *Psychosomatic Methods in Painless Childbirth* (New York: Pergamon Press, 1959).
5. Hans Selye, *Stress of Life* (New York: McGraw-Hill, 1956).
6. Hans Selye, "The Stress Syndrome," in Jeannette R. Folta and Edith S. Deck, eds., *A Sociological Framework for Patient Care* (New York: John Wiley, 1966, pp. 253–257).
7. Hans Selye, interviewed by Laurence Cherry, "On the Real Benefits of Eustress," *Psychology Today,* March 1978, pp. 60–63, 69–70.
8. Mary Irene Crawford, "Physiological and Behavioral Cues to Disturbances in Childbirth" (Doctoral diss., Teachers College, Columbia University, 1968).

process? Of course, but of itself, it is a stressful process, the stress of which is intensified by anxiety. It is not so much the process of stress that is relevant to childbirth education but the process of coping with stress—adaptation.

SELYE'S THEORY AND CHILDBIRTH EDUCATION

Among the theories of stress and adaptation, Hans Selye's is particularly relevant to understanding the functioning of the human body in its attempts to cope during stress.[9] Although Selye's clinical experiments have dealt primarily with cardiac patients, in a discussion of the application of his theories to childbirth education he agreed that there was no fault in the logic that interprets preparation for childbearing as a form of stress adaptation.[10]

According to Selye, human beings exist simultaneously on three interrelated planes—the ①biological, or structural; the ②physiological, or functional; and the ③psychological, or mental (Fig. 2–1). Any change in the state of one of these planes will result in a change in the other two. For example, Crawford describes the situation of the laboring woman. When the woman's anxiety increases (psychological plane), the adrenal glands secrete hormones (physiological plane), which suppress uterine muscle contraction (biological plane).[5]

This same triplanal model can be used to view the expectant mother. The expectant mother also exists simultaneously on the three planes, biological, physiological and psychological. It is the goal of childbirth education to provide the mother, in a manner that she can absorb, with the mechanisms by which she can cope with the stresses of labor and delivery before finding herself in the unalterable situation of labor.

As described previously, three components to the process of childbirth education have been consistently identified—providing adequate facts, controlled relaxation, and specific learned breathing techniques. Applying Selye's theory to this process, the manner of adaptation becomes obvious.

Facts Lead to Sense of Control

The first step in the preparation is to provide accurate, adequate facts about the labor and delivery process and the attending events to be expected upon

9. Hans Selye, "The Stress Syndrome," p. 256.
10. Hans Selye, personal interview, University of Montreal, February 18, 1972.

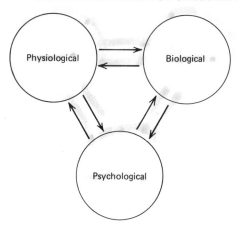

Figure 2–1.

Selye's three intercommunicating planes. Hans Selye's stress theory provides an excellent framework for unifying the process of childbirth education. By expanding the concept of education beyond the purely cognitive domain, it becomes possible to view childbearing and the birth process as it effects the total person—biologically, physiologically, and psychologically.

admission to the hospital. This component serves to lessen anxiety about the unknown and create a positive mental attitude toward the experience. It also helps the woman (and her partner) to be able to relate the relaxation and breathing techniques to the labor process. Psychologically this understanding lends predictability to the situation and provides a sense of control in a situation that most people anticipate as one in which they will lose control.[11]

Exercises to Prepare

The second step in preparing the expectant mother to cope with labor and delivery is to present a regular program of exercise. In this program two kinds of exercises play a part. While the exercises are different in nature, there is an underlying commonality in their purpose of stress adaptation. The first set of exercises, sometimes referred to as body building or physical fitness exercises, are preliminary to the controlled relaxation, which is usually considered the key to prepared childbirth. These exercises do prepare the body; however, it

11. Betty L. Highley and Ramona T. Mercer, "Safeguarding the Laboring Woman's Sense of Control," *American Journal of Maternal-Child Nursing*, Jan/Feb, 1978, p. 39.

is not only the stretching and exercising of muscles that is important. The act of exercising is the real preconditioner. Labor is a process of progressive muscular contractions. Because labor is a prolonged muscular activity, the contractions themselves become stressors eliciting body reactions to cope with the stress. By engaging in regular daily sessions of mild exercise up to the time of labor, the woman prepares her body to respond to the stressors of labor by developing specific responses to the stressor "muscular activity" and is better able to cope with this stressor during the actual labor process. This explanation involves the somaphysiology or body functioning.

Exercises for Self-Help

The second set of exercises, which are more often associated with prepared childbirth, involve the neuromuscular control exercises. They are designed to develop a specific learned response to relax groups of muscles SELECTIVELY. Selective muscular relaxation during stress is a conscious mechanism for minimizing stress caused by loss of control, anxiety and intensified perception of pain. The conscious attempt to relax all muscles not in use provides a focal point for attention. It is thought that neurologically reciprocal inhibition alters the person's perception,[12] that is, the harder she concentrates on relaxing, the less she is aware of the pains of the sensations of the concentration. Conversely, the less she concentrates, the more she is aware of painful sensations. In addition to providing a focal point, the controlled relaxation activities during labor help the woman to conserve energy and prevent the physiologic–psychologic irritability that results from structural fatigue.

Complex Activities Increase Concentration

The third step in preparing expectant parents to cope with the stress of labor and delivery is to provide specific complex patterns of behavior to use in response to the actual sensations perceived during labor contractions. The complex activity involves controlled relaxation combined with controlled breathing and massage combinations. The woman is taught to use techniques in response to what she feels—to use the less complex patterns for as long as they work to keep her comfortable. She is not trying to ignore the contraction nor is she trying to dissociate her mind from it. Rather, she is focusing on response to the sensations instead of the stimulus of the sensations themselves. Pain perception can be altered greatly by conscious specific activities

12.   Lamaze, *op. cit.*, p. 45.

as a means of coping rather than the more commonly seen "fight or flight" reaction in the untrained woman. In addition to altering pain perception, by responding deliberately to each contraction with a learned behavior, the woman is able to enjoy a sense of having some control of her own body and its reactions, a feeling that enhances self-confidence and satisfaction with the experience.

Preparation Leads to Stress Adaptation

The total effect of preparation is to provide coping mechanisms on all three planes. Psychologically, the woman who has specific activities to work with in her labor has a positive outlook. Her husband, acting as labor coach, serves to validate her efforts by providing a direct link with the preparation classes through his observations and communication during labor and is a source of emotional support in her efforts to work with her labor. Physiologically, the woman is less anxious, less likely to hyperventilate without detection, and more apt to conserve energy and minimize her overall body needs for oxygen. Biologically, the woman is more likely to be positioned comfortably or amenable to changes in position because of the information gained in the classes regarding anatomy and physiology of labor and particular comfort measures taught to the husband as coach.

To summarize, the common elements of the process of childbirth education are correct information, controlled relaxation, and deliberate learned behavior patterns in response to labor contractions. These elements interact with the already intercommunicating planes of structural, functional, and psychological existence to permit the laboring woman with the assistance of her labor coach husband to confidently and intelligently cooperate with the obstetrical staff and thereby reduce the stresses of labor to a manageable level.

CHILDBIRTH EDUCATION AND CRISIS INTERVENTION

In addition to the support for this explanation in stress theory, the literature on crisis intervention also provides a basis for childbirth education in many forms.[13,14] Pregnancy and birth, although very normal aspects of human life,

13.   Donna C. Aguilera, Janice M. Messick, and Marlene S. Farrell, *Crisis Intervention: Theory and Methodology* (St. Louis: C. V. Mosby, 1970).
14.   Paul H. Glaser and Lois N. Glaser, eds., *Families in Crisis* (New York: Harper & Row, 1970).

are also pivotal points for family development. The status of the family structure is altered by the potential and later real introduction of another member. This disruption has been identified as one of the maturational crises of the life cycle. LeMasters in particular discusses the very real crisis that occurs when the romanticized concept of parenthood comes into conflict with the reality of parenthood.[15] In our society, this particular problem occurs because there is little opportunity for expectant parents to have experienced prolonged contact with infants or young children. The situation is further compounded by the nomadic nature of today's young adults who are usually a far distance from or completely separated from the older members of their family of orientation. Where in the past, young adults turned for guidance to parents, grandparents, or older aunts or uncles living under the same roof, today's expectant parents most frequently live by themselves with no easy access to the older generation and must rely on other sources for their support and information. Other young parents, mass media, and health professionals have been thrust into the role of providing what had been an intrafamilial service in past generations.

Childbirth education, therefore, takes on another dimension when one perceives the need to assist expectant parents in developing their coping mechanisms so that they will be able to resolve the maturational crisis of childbearing in adaptive rather than maladaptive ways. Childbirth education encompasses a very short span of time in the life of a family. It can be a crucial factor, however, in the ease with which the expectant parents can assume their parental roles. And, it is more often the affective rather than the cognitive aspects of the childbirth education experience that will influence the outcomes. Therefore, it is again the process of childbirth education rather than the content that grows out of the theory as an explanation of the phenomenon.

Education for the Future

Correct information about "life with baby" is essential. Many parents go through an entire pregnancy without giving any consideration to the real changes that may occur in their life style because of a baby. Romantic ideals of babyhood and myths about parenthood, especially motherliness, provide parents with a mental set of expectations that no normal newborn infant can fulfill. Discussions about normal newborn behavior with groups of expectant

15. E. E. LeMasters, "Parenthood as Crisis," in Marvin B. Sussman, ed., *Sourcebook in Marriage and the Family*, 2nd ed. (Boston: Houghton-Mifflin, 1963), p. 197.

parents afford the opportunity to dispel some of the myths as well as to encourage individual parents to translate generalizations into personal terms, and, perhaps for the first time, assist parents to think about what it will be like to bring a totally dependent stranger into their lives. These kinds of discussions also help parents to understand that they should not expect to like their child all the time, that parents are not always perfect, that mother-love is not always an instantaneous happening occurring from the moment of birth, and that every baby, like every adult, will have a unique personality that makes him different from every other baby while his babyhood will progress in predictable patterns. The reassurances drawn out of parent-to-parent discussions allay some of the natural fears and later forestall unnecessary self-castigation for what are essentially normal feelings and reactions in the parents themselves.

Improving Self Confidence

Another affective benefit from the process of prepared childbearing is a result of the total experience. Parents who make an effort to correct deficiencies that they have recognized in their own knowledge of birth, who seek to help themselves as much as possible during the birthing process and who are able to emerge from the experience of bringing their child into the world with a sense of dignity and a feeling of control of the situation carry with them an aura of confidence through to the puerperal period. Self-confidence through accomplishment leads to further faith in one's ability to handle other situations, namely the care of the baby.[16] This sequence of events is enhanced by the early achievement of the first tasks of parenting. Parents who are able to see their child at birth are immediately able to recognize and accept that baby as their own and to verify that it is whole and undamaged and to establish the sex of the infant. Accomplishing this task at birth allows the parents to move on to the next tasks of learning the uniqueness of their child and practicing some of the caring skills.

Self-confidence and self-reliability are truly the goals of childbirth education. While the focus of content is most often emphasizing the elements of the most imminent threat—labor and delivery—the intent of the process is to assist expectant parents in moving comfortably into their new roles as parents. Comfortable parents can rely on their own judgment in day-to-day matters and are confident in their daily decisions.

16.   Jeannette L. Sasmor, "The Effects of Prepared Childbirth on the Early Establishment of a Healthy Maternal-Child Relationship" (Paper presented to Thirteenth International Congress of Pediatrics, Vienna, Austria, Sept., 1971).

CHILDBIRTH EDUCATION: ADULT EDUCATION

The final theoretical framework for discussing childbirth education is found in the work of Malcolm Knowles and his interpretation of androgogy, or adult education.[17] Knowles maintains that adults learn in ways that are different from those in which children learn. However, most education experiences are planned on pedagogical principles, which do not take into consideration that adults are older, more experienced, and learn differently than do children. In planning for childbirth education programs one must plan for androgogical experiences. To do this, it is essential that one first accept the basic assumption that teachers and learners are adults engaging in an interactive process.[18] The word, "interactive" is the key. It implies that both teacher and learner are each sending and receiving messages; there is communication in both directions. Second, it implies that both teacher and learner have something to contribute to the exchange; that no one person is the undisputed fountain of wisdom.

Characteristics of Adult Learners

Gorman has identified several characteristics of adults interacting in learning situations that have particular relevance for childbirth education planners.[19]

1. Learners and teachers bring with them to the classroom a cluster of understandings, skills, appreciations, attitudes, and feelings that have personal meaning to them and are in effect the sum of their reactions to previous stimuli
Styles of teaching and styles of learning are evidence of individual prior experience with education. But, in addition, every adult in the childbirth education class carries a wealth of background, sometimes accurate, sometimes myth, about the childbearing process. Expectant parents select specific courses for reasons known only to them; teachers become committed to certain courses for reasons that stem from their own experiences. It is the covert motivation of learner and teacher that frequently enters the courses as a "hidden agenda" to be alluded to and dealt with indirectly over the duration of a course.

17.   Malcom Knowles, ed., *Handbook of Adult in the United States* (Washington: Adult Education Association, 1960).
18.   Alfred H. Gorman, *Teachers and Learners: The Interactive Process of Education* (Boston: Allyn & Bacon, 1969).
19.   *Ibid.*

2. Learners and teachers are individually different in many ways when grouped according to ability
Despite the fact that every member of an expectant parents' class will be a parent within a given span of time, each expectant parent in the class is unique, a culmination of all the prior experiences that that person has had. Sharing of varying points of view and ideas, exchanging opinions, clarifying questions can be an enriching experience for a group of people who all share a common characteristic—a soon-to-be over pregnancy.

3. Learners and teachers have a developed concept of self, which directly affects their behavior
Teaching styles are so obviously an outgrowth of one's self-concept, where rigidity or flexibility are the outward signs of the inward concept and security. Learning styles are also a manifestation of self-concept. It is fairly easy to get lost in a large lecture section in which participation is measured by the quantity of notes taken. It is much more difficult to be an active participant in a small group of people in which discussion is the teaching method when one's self-concept does not permit openness or frankness. It is important that people be allowed to remain private if they choose. Quietness in a discussion group does not mean lack of learning.

4. Learning may be defined as a change in behavior
If this definition of learning is accepted, then all planning for learning in the childbirth education sphere must include identification of the desired change in behavior, a specified means for attaining that change, criteria for determining if the change has been attained, and a system for carrying out the plan that includes all aspects of the plan.

5. Learning requires activity on the part of the learner. He must not be passive
All presentation of material must be made in a way that will cause the learner to think—to answer questions posed mentally, to relate the material to individual situations, to picture graphic examples. It is obvious that straight lecture is the least desirable way of achieving learner activity, although it can be done skillfully even in large groups by creative teachers.

6. Learners learn what THEY actively desire to learn. They do not learn what they do not accept or come to accept
Selective attention is a big part of the learning situation for expectant parents. Anxieties about the labor, the condition of the baby, even about survival through the birth itself are distorters for many parents. Similarly, prejudice for or against medication, for or against breast-feeding, or any other emotionally

laden subject will frequently interfere overtly or covertly with the learning process in the childbirth education class. It is to the benefit of the teaching–learning process to spend some time discovering the learners' goals and objectives for any particular childbirth education course.

7. Learning is enhanced when learners accept responsibility for their own learning
This concept is perhaps one of the significant differences between traditional learning situations and those planned for adults. The idea of the learner being responsible for his own learning is foreign to most people—teachers and learners alike. It changes the role of the teacher from that of wisdom-giver to that of motivator and facilitator. In childbirth education, this idea of learner-responsibility is particularly important because the successful use of the psychomotor aspects of the preparation depend heavily on the habituation of them that results from regular practice. Practice, in turn, depends on the willingness of the participant to assume responsibility for actually carrying out the out-of-class activities. It, therefore, becomes part of the teaching role to help the learner accept that responsibility.

8. Learning is influenced by physical and social environment
Childbirth education as a mass movement got its start in the homey surroundings of the living room of the childbirth educator. Frequently, this meant interruptions by the educator's family in the classes as well as disruption in the family life of the educator caused by the imposition of an educational situation on the home situation at regular intervals. Many experienced childbirth educators gradually learned that this was a less than ideal physical setting and relocated the classes to more educationally conducive environments such as community centers, local hospitals, and junior colleges. In the case of the social environment, group discussions and other kinds of activities have long been considered desirable as a climate for parent education.

9. Learning occurs on successively deeper levels
This axiom refers back to finding out the learner's goals and proceeding with that point in mind. This is not a new idea as teachers have long operated on a principle of teaching cognitive skills by moving from the known to the unknown.

10. Learning is deepened when the learning situation provides opportunity for applying learning in as realistic a situation as is feasible
This belief is a strong factor in planning teaching strategies that will allow the learners to visualize exactly what can be expected—environment, procedures, process of labor, care of newborn, parental response—and in selecting

the location for the classes. Although not always feasible, it is desirable that childbirth education classes he held in the hospital in which the parents will deliver. Familiarity with the hospital environment serves to some extent to desensitize the parents, bringing them to a greater level of comfort than is possible if they are able to avoid the situation until they are already stressed by labor. Secondly, it helps them to think through the class material within the context in which they have to actually carry it out.

11. Learners are motivated when they understand and accept the purposes of the learning situation
The days of the physician saying "Just don't worry, I'll take care of everything" are definitely numbered. Intelligent consumerism in health care is slowly becoming a reality. A part of being an intelligent consumer is the need to know.

12. Learners are motivated by successful experiences
Similar to the idea of moving from the known to the unknown is the idea of planning experiences that move from the simple to the complex. This concept is really a building block theory that permits the learner to demonstrate competence in a simple skill, incorporate that skill, and add another to it so that the end result is very complex behavior. Success needs to be built into the learning situation through planned learning sequences and a teaching–student feedback system that keeps the student informed of successful progress.

13. Learners are motivated by teacher acceptance
The interpersonal aspects of childbirth education are indeed the key to learner satisfaction. Individual uniqueness and individual worth are two concepts that the childbirth educator must accept in order to be able to accept each learner and to assist that learner in exploring his or her own hidden agenda for the classes.

14. Learners are motivated when they can associate new learning with previous learning
This concept goes one step further than just accepting each learner. It suggests that the teacher encourage each learner to share his or her prior experiences that relate to the topics at hand. This is a definitely useful tool for expectant parents as it helps them individually to relate content in their own individual terms to their lives and it encourages a sharing of ideas and experiences, which frequently turn out to be shared commonly by expectant parents. This latter process is often the only normative data that many of the parents have about the experience of pregnancy.

15. *Learners are motivated when they can see the usefulness of the learning in their own personal terms*

Since no one can reverse the process of pregnancy and birth short of termination, the imminent goal of labor and delivery makes parents attending childbirth education classes a group whose motivation to learn is probably higher than average. As the birth date draws closer, gnawing anxiety grows. Expectant parents are grateful for any and all information they can glean before the event. How they use that information will be determined by their own goals for the type of experience they want to have.

Gorman's characteristics are one attempt to describe teachers and learners. There are many others, but the framework of looking at the teaching–learning process as an interactive process is by far the most meaningful for childbirth education, which is extremely short and depends heavily on the affective domain to accomplish the major part of its educational goals.

COMMUNICATION COMPETENCE

Effective communication is the means of achieving the goals of childbirth education. It requires that the teacher understand the theoretical basis for the process of childbirth education, the nature of the modern expectant parent's maturational development, and the characteristics of the teacher and learners in adult education. Further, for the teacher to be an effective communicator, he or she must be aware of his or her current ability to communicate. Borman and colleagues have identified levels of competence in communication that are definitely relevant to childbirth education[20] (Fig. 2–2).

Unconscious Incompetence

The childbirth educator who is *unconsciously incompetent* is unable to communicate effectively but does not recognize that this is a personal failure. The failure may stem from having identified objectives that are inappropriate or unrealistic for the learner or from sending messages that are not understandable to the learner, or from an inability to listen and respond appropriately to the learner, or from body language that is disturbing to those who are trying to learn. The unconsciously incompetent childbirth educator accepts no respon-

20. Ernest Borman, et al., *The Modern Organization* (Englewood Cliffs, NJ, Prentice-Hall, 1969), pp. 131–35.

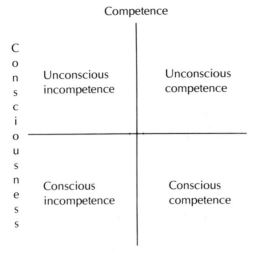

Figure 2-2.

People constantly move from one quadrant to the other depending on many factors. Conscious competence is the most productive mode.

siblity for the breakdown in communication but rather blames the breakdown on learner inabilities such as lack of intelligence or motivation.

Conscious Incompetence

Conscious incompetence is not unusual when a competent nurse is suddenly thrust into the role of childbirth educator. This situation occurs frequently because teaching parents' classes is often looked upon as a rewarding situation and used as such. However, even an excellent postpartum nurse is not necessarily a competent childbirth educator. This person is aware of such incompetence and how that awareness is handled will depend on the options that are open. But the most useful approach is to take action that will move the educator from incompetence to competence, that is, seeking adequate preparation to move into a teaching role.

Unconscious Competence

The childbirth educator who is *unconsciously competent* is able to teach effectively but is unaware of how he or she is able to do it. This person has cultivated the communication skills that have worked in the past and carries them out automatically. It is often developed by frequent repetition. For the childbirth educator, frequent repetition means regular presentation of the same lesson plan without variation, over and over. In most instances this repetition works and is very effective, because the situation allows this lack of alteration. However, not all teaching situations are the same even though the content may be similar. The person who is unconsciously competent is unable to adapt to changes and may be forced by change of class circumstances to perform incompetently, either consciously or unconsciously.

Conscious Competence

The childbirth educator who is *consciously competent* is able to be flexible because of an awareness of factors that influence human communication, a sensitivity to verbal and nonverbal messages sent by the learner, and the ability to adapt teaching activities to the needs of the learning group, which is a part of being totally comfortable with the content matter, so that necessary changes do not alter learning objectives but can be worked in around them. In other words, the *consciously* competent childbirth educator knows what is being taught, how it is being taught, and why it works. Effective communication is the means of achieving the goals of childbirth education. It is essential that childbirth educators strive to function at the level of conscious competence. This type of functioning requires not only superficial self-awareness but continual planning and evaluation of both the product of childbirth education—the expectant parents' experiences—and the process of childbirth education—the teacher and teaching situation. If one removes the pass–fail connotation from the process of evaluation and looks upon it as a means of gathering information to use for making decisions about how to teach, perhaps all childbirth educators could comfortably build the process of evaluation into the childbirth education overall plan. For it is only by review and evaluation that high quality can be an achievable goal.

SUMMARY

The theoretical framework for childbirth education discussed in this chapter finds its basis in the theories of stress adaptation and crisis intervention. The process of childbirth education provides expectant parents with adaptive kinds of behavior with which they can deal with the stresses of labor. By providing this preparation before labor, this form of anticipatory guidance assists parents to move through the maturational crisis anticipated by the life-cycle highlight of childbearing. This basis for content is augmented by adult learinig theory and communication theory which, when combined, provide the modes for teaching strategies that make childbirth education an indentifiable entity.

BIBLIOGRAPHY

Anthony EJ, Benedek T: *Parenthood, Its Psychology and Psychopathology.* Boston, Little, Brown & Co, 1970.

Baird S: Crisis Intervention Theory is Maternal-Infant Nursing. *JOGN* **5:**1, Jan/Feb 1976.

Balderstone J: Romance, Marriage and Parenthood. *American Baby,* Dec 1973.

Bruce S: Do Prenatal Programs Really Prepare for Parenthood? *Hospital Topics,* Nov 1965.

Cassidy J: A Nurse Looks at Childbirth Anxiety. *JOGN* **3:**1, Jan/Feb 1974.

Cohen A: *Childbirth Is Ecstasy.* San Francisco, Aquarus Publishing Co, 1971.

Colman A, Colman L: *Pregnancy: The Psychological Experience.* New York, Herder and Jerder, 1971.

Donner G: Parenthood a Crisis: A Role for the Psychiatric Nurse. *Perspectives in Psychiatric Care* **1:**2, 1972.

Dzik RS: Transactional Analysis, Crisis Intervention. *JOGN* **5:**1, Jan/Feb 1976.

Griffith S: Pregnancy As an Event with Crisis Potential for Marital Partners: A Summary of A Study of Interpersonal Needs. *JOGN* **5:**6, Nov/Dec 1976.

Hobbs D: Parenthood as Crisis: A Third Study. *Journal of Marriage and the Family,* March 1963.

Larsen V: The Stresses of the Childbearing Years. *The Am J of PH,* LVI, Jan 1966.

LeMasters EE: *Parents in Modern America.* Homewood, Ill, The Dorsey Press, 1970.

Levi L: *Stress: Source, Management, Prevention.* New York, Liveright Publishing Corp, 1967.

McQuade W, Aikmon A: *Stress.* New York, Bantam Books, 1977.

Parad, HJ: *Crisis Intervention: Selected Readings.* New York, Family Services Association, 1965.

Selye H: *Stress of Life,* rev. New York, McGraw-Hill, 1976.

Selye H: *Stress Without Distress.* Philadelphia, J.B. Lippincott, 1974.

Selye H: *The Stress of My Life.* Toronto, McClelland and Stewart, 1977.

Tanzer D: *Why Natural Childbirth?* Garden City, New York Doubleday & Co, 1972.

Willmuth LR: Prepared Childbirth and the Concept of Control. *Journal OB/GYN Neonatal Nursing* **4:**5, Sept/Oct 1975.

Chapter **3**

Self-Help Approaches for Parents During Labor

The specific content of a childbirth education course will depend largely on the particular goal of the course and the course objectives (Chapter 4). Most childbirth education courses with the goal of preparing parents for controlled labor fall into one of three schools of approach to psychoprophylaxis: Read, Lamaze, or Eclectic.

This chapter will describe each of the approaches and its philosophy and techniques as they are taught to parents. The value in knowing the differences among approaches is that it permits the nurse to support the parents' efforts, regardless of which school they follow. This support may be sought in the labor situation or it may be that the nurse is regarded as a resource person in the local community and parents seek the nurse's advice about what they are learning. If the nurse is knowledgeable about a particular approach, it gives credibility to what they are doing and will reinforce their motivation.[1,2]

READ METHOD—CHILDBIRTH WITHOUT FEAR

The writings of Dr. Grantly Dick-Read were to fire the minds of millions of people around the world. Yet, by his own report his writings were scoffed at

1.   Jeannette L. Sasmor, Constance Castor, and Patricia Hassid, "The Childbirth Team During Labor," *American Journal of Nursing,* March 1973.
2.   Patricia Huprich, "Assisting the Couple Through a Lamaze Labor and Delivery," *American Journal of Maternal-Child Nursing,* July/August 1977, p. 245.

by his own colleagues when they initially appeared.[3] Read first experienced the possibility of unmedicated childbirth while attending a poor woman delivering at home. It was the first time in his experience that a woman refused medication (at that time chloroform). After the delivery, he asked her why she had refused to which she responded with a fateful question: "It didn't hurt. It wasn't meant to, was it, doctor?" Through thirty years of practice, Dr. Read was to ponder this question, only to answer in his own mind, "No. It was not meant to."[4]

Read's own words describe his philosophy better than any interpretation could. The following quotation states his theory of what he called natural childbirth:

> Superstition, civilization and culture have brought influences to bear upon the minds of women which have introduced justifiable fears and anxieties concerning labor. The more cultured the races of the earth [sic] have become, so much more positive have they been in pronouncing childbirth to be a painful and dangerous ordeal. Thus fear and anticipation of pain have given rise to natural protective tensions in the body, and such tensions are not of the mind only, for the mechanisms of the protective actions by the body includes muscle tension. Unfortunately, the natural tension produced by fear influences those muscles which close the womb and oppose the dilatation of the birth canal during labor. Therefore, fear inhibits, that is to say, gives rise to resistance at the outlet of the womb, when in the normal state those muscles should be relaxed and free from tension. This resistance gives rise to pain because the uterus is supplied with sensitive nerve endings which record pain arising from excessive tension. Therefore, fear, tension, and pain are three veils opposed to the natural design which have been concerned with preparation for and attendance at childbirth. If fear, tension and pain go hand in hand, then it must be necessary to relieve tension and to overcome fear in order to eliminate pain. The implementation of my theory demonstrates the methods by which fear may be overcome, tension may be eliminated and replaced by physical and mental relaxation.[5]

From this philosophy, Read went on to identify what he refers to as factors that predispose to a low threshold of pain interpretation. It is the clear

3. Grantly Dick-Read, *Childbirth Without Fear,* 2nd ed. (New York: Harper & Row, 1959), p. 39–40.
4. *Ibid.*
5. *Ibid.*

identification of these eight factors that serve as a basis for the education and training commonly called the Read method.

Read's Pain Intensifiers

Read perceived the mind and body as an interacting whole. Thus his fear–tension–pain cycle is an extension of this idea. It was his belief that there were identifiable conditions that could either be avoided or treated, conditions that could influence the course of labor if they persisted.[6]

1. Anemia: Read attributes to neurologist Henry Head the observation that diminished general resistance to pain can be caused by anemia. Although physiological anemia is a normal occurrence with the hypervolemia of pregnancy, Read observed that if the woman reports tiredness, exhaustion after normal activities, breathlessness for which she can find no cause, depression, and loss of appetite, she will shortly run out of the endurance necessary to cope with the stresses of labor.

2. Tiredness of Body: Whether a woman starts labor exhausted or expends large amounts of energy, physical and emotional, during labor, as labor progresses she will be less able to cope and more susceptible to the increasing sensations.

3. Weariness of Mind: In this category, Read refers especially to the atmosphere in which the woman must labor. He maintains that overstimulation from any sensory source will interfere with the woman's ability to cope mentally and thereby intensify her discomforts.

4. Depression and disappointment: Read also attributes this intensifier to the atmosphere of the labor situation. During the seemingly unending repetition of contractions the woman's resources are eroded. Read blames loneliness and ignorance for the woman who becomes depressed or disappointed with her progress. For the loneliness and ignorance, he holds the attendants totally responsible.

5. Loss of control: When the woman loses her sense of control, she is subject to intensified response to all stimuli.

6. Centralization of thought: Focusing all one's attention on the sensation of the contraction, its cause and results, will invariably intensify the perception of the sensation.

7. Autosuggestion: The role of autosuggestion is partly a direct result of past experience or stores of memory impressions in the unconscious. This stored memory may be from direct experience or from hearsay. Because pain

6. *Ibid.*

is a subjective experience, when contractions begin, the personal memory impressions are called into play and will have a direct effect on the woman's pain perception.

8. Suggestion: Unlike autosuggestion, which is generated by the woman, suggestion is produced by the people around her. In addition to what the woman has heard from her mother or girlfriends about the painfulness of contractions, she will unconsciously receive impressions from the attitudes of the labor attendants, from facial expression or questions, from the very atmosphere of surgical asepsis and the possibility of surgical intervention. Thus, she will anticipate painful sensation.

Read and Relaxation

As a result of his perception of the mind–body mutuality, Read spends as much time considering ways to relax the mind as he does advocating techniques for relaxing the body. He believes that the vast majority of women carry images in their minds about childbearing. Some of these images are a part of their own fantasies surrounding the growth and development of the baby, but, a large portion of the images are learned as part of their cultural heritage. This heritage stretches from the time of the Bible to modern-day communications, television, and films. Not least as a source of information are relatives and friends, many of whom are as ignorant about the physiological process of birth as the woman herself.

Read and Education

Read recognized the crying need for adequate education during the antepartal period. These three principles guided him in caring for pregnant women:

> The first principle is to insure good health, both physical and mental, during pregnancy, and so minimizing the discomforts of labor and necessity for interference. Secondly, we desire that childbirth should be accompanied by a sense of maternal achievement and satisfaction, and that the mother–child relationship should be enhanced by pride and pleasure and not tainted by resentment or distressing memories. And, thirdly, that the mother should desire and be willing to have more children because of, not in spite of, her experience of childbirth.

To carry out these principles, Read identified five objectives of good prenatal care, the first two for the physician and the last three for the woman:

1. To observe the physical condition of pregnant women in order to prevent or diagnose as early as possible any abnormalities or irregularities that may disturb the health of either the mother or child during pregnancy, parturition, or the puerperium.
2. To be forewarned of physical or mechanical factors predisposing to a difficult labor, in order to avoid as far as possible emergent and unpremeditated interference.
3. To educate pregnant women so that the inhibiting influence of fear may be replaced by understanding and confidence.
4. To instruct women in the phenomenon of labor so that they may interpret its varying sensations correctly and meet its demands with discernment, patience, and self-control in order that they may assist the natural forces and not resist them.
5. To teach women how to prepare themselves for the birth of the child in a manner that still enables them:
   a. to relax when tension will cause resistance and pain, particularly during the inactivity of the first stage of labor;
   b. to have control of respiration so that they can breathe deeply, rapidly, or quietly when requested or to hold the breath when called upon to do so by the attendant;
   c. to be physically fit to persist in the expulsive effort of the second stage of labor, without undue exhaustion.

Adequate education during the prenatal period is the keystone of the Read Method. Dispelling myths and providing accurate, easy-to-understand information about the process of labor and delivery return childbearing to the realm of a physiological function, a normal aspect of human life. Hygiene and nutrition are also an important part of Read preparation because the emphasis is on having the healthiest woman possible arrive in labor. All these add immeasurably to the mental relaxation or calmness that is so important to the attitude of the woman as she approaches the labor experience.

Physical relaxation is equally important and can be accomplished readily when the mind is relaxed and free from unwarranted fears and anxieties. In fact, physical relaxation and mental relaxation go hand in hand. Given adequate information to overcome fear bred of ignorance, the woman who can relax completely, that is, who can reduce muscular tension to an absolute minimum, will find that her mental activity will also slow down to a minimum. Many women who can completely relax drift off into a natural deep sleep.

Learning to Relax

The position recommended for relaxation is usually right lateral or left lateral because it becomes increasingly difficult for the woman to lie on her back in late pregnancy. Relaxation practice during pregnancy follows a usual pattern. Because regular slow breathing has a calming effect itself, it is combined with the efforts to relax. These exercises attempt to help the woman to identify tension and relaxation. Lying comfortably on her side with a pillow supporting her shoulders and upper leg, the woman is told to "Take a deep breath through an open mouth; curl up the toes and tense the muscles of one leg (pause). Release the breath slowly and relax the whole limb." This exercise is repeated until the woman has tensed and relaxed all the voluntary muscle groups. She is asked each time to compare in her own mind the tension and relaxation so that she can distinguish the sensations. After the exercises a session of relaxation demonstration is held. In a warm room that has been darkened, the woman is asked to lie in a comfortable position. If she is cold, she is covered with a blanket. She is then to relax to the best of her ability. A session might last for 15 to 30 minutes. During that time, the woman who has mastered complete relaxation usually drifts off to sleep. She may merely become sleepy, exhibiting signs of incomplete relaxation such as irregularity of breathing, flickering of eyelids, eye movement, shifting of fingers or toes, or uncontrollable swallowings. Response to external stimuli such as sudden noises is also a sign of residual tension. Usually with practice, most people can overcome residual tension.

Read And Breathing Techniques

The use of breathing techniques seems to be a necessary corollary to the use of relaxation to reduce tension and maintain a calm environment for the mother and baby. Read recommends essentially three techniques: Deep breathing both in abdominal respirations and thoracic respiration, shallow breathing, and breath-holding for the second stage.

In teaching the breathing techniques, the Read Method combines the breathing techniques with physical fitness exercises that serve their own good purpose in readying the woman's body for delivery. There are seven combinations of physical fitness and breathing exercises that are an integral part of the preparation of the woman. The six breathing exercises are shown in Figures 3-1 through 3-6.

Exercise 7 is a muscle control exercise and consists of the following steps:

1. Concentrate on the anus.
2. Close the anus firmly until it feels as though it is being drawn up into the rectum. (Continued on page 35)

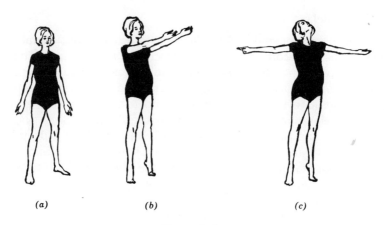

(a)   (b)   (c)

Figure 3-1.

(a) Standing on a broad comfortable base, hands at sides, palms forward . . .
(b) . . . raise hands in front of body as high as the shoulder . . . (c) . . . taking in
a long, slow deep breath, swing the arms outward, dropping head backward slightly.
Allow breath to release slowly as body returns to starting position. Repeat 6 times.

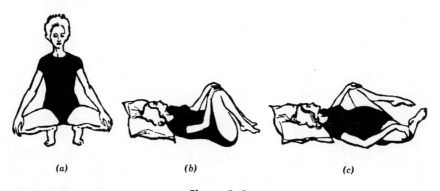

(a)   (b)   (c)

Figure 3-2.

(a) Standing with a straight back, raise up on toes and lower body to squatting
position. Place hands on knees and push legs as far apart as possible keeping back
straight. Rise to standing position, lowering heels to ground last. Repeat 5 times.
(b) Alternative for the woman who is not able to maintain balance for squatting.
Lying comfortably with shoulders and head supported, and both hips touching the
ground, raise both knees as close to chest as possible . . . (c) . . . allow knees to
fall apart sideways, place hands on knees and exert continuous pressure to press
them as widely apart as possible. Repeat 5 times.

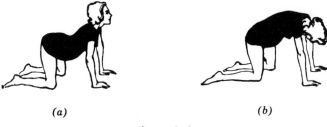

Figure 3-3.

(a) Getting down on hands and knees with hands about the level of the shoulders and shoulder width apart, knees about 8 inches apart, back hollow and arms slightly bent, take a deep breath . . . (b) . . . drop head forward, straighten arms, raise back and move buttocks inward letting breath out as back is arching. Return to starting position. Repeat 6 times.

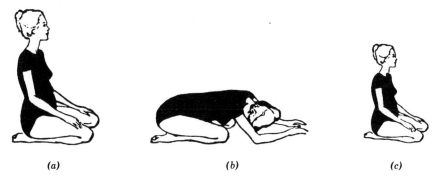

Figure 3-4.

(a) With back straight, sit on heels with legs flexed under body and hands on knees which are about 12 inches apart . . . (b) . . . keeping back straight, take in a deep breath, leaning forward until elbows and arms are flat on the floor in front of knees while exhaling . . . (c) . . . take another deep breath as body is raised again. When upright, press hands on knees, hollow back, and raise the chin. Repeat 8 times.

3. Keep the legs and buttocks as relaxed as possible.
4. Hold the anus tight for a definite pause.
5. Repeat twelve times twice a day.

   These exercises are taught during the prenatal period and practiced regularly up to the time of delivery. They are as important to the woman as the relaxation training and factual education.

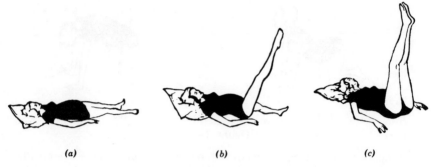

(a)   (b)   (c)

Figure 3–5.

(a) Lying on back, raise right leg as high as is comfortable without flexing knee. Keep foot relaxed breathing in as leg is raised . . . (b) . . . slowly lower leg to floor while exhaling. Do not point toe. Repeat with left leg. Repeat entire sequence for both legs 6 times. (c) Variation. Lying on back, raise both legs as high as is comfortable, breathing in as the legs are raised. Lower legs slowly to ground while exhaling. This exercise is much more useful to the woman postpartally as a strengthener for flabby abdominal muscles.

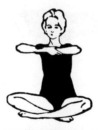

Figure 3–6.

Take a deep breath, hold, grasp both wrists in opposite hands, pushing skin up forearm. Relax and repeat. Breath should be held for a count of 10 arm pushes. Gradually this can be increased until breath can be held for a count of 20 or about 20 seconds.

Read on Medication

Despite the fact that Read abhors indiscriminate use of obstetrical analgesia and anesthesia, his followers' interpretation of natural childbirth as total lack of medication is not quite accurate. Read himself said, "The origin of this damaging myth is of long standing, although only recently brought to my notice by a doctor whose wife wanted me to attend her. He had read a book in the medical library in which it states that I do not give anesthetics. I knew at once the book to which he referred. It is popular with medical students as it is short and easy to read. This inaccuracy persists, uncorrected by the author, who has been fully aware that it is untrue for at least ten years!"[7]

In fact, quite to the contrary, Read has stated three rules on the use of analgesia:

1. No woman in labor should be allowed to suffer pain.
2. Analgesics are always available by the bedside for the woman to use herself if and when she desires to do so.
3. Analgesics are given as a drug or inhalant according to the clinical indication and judgment of the attendant.

He goes on to state, however, that "no anesthetic is accepted when offered, by the majority of women so educated." He then supports this belief with the understanding that the women must be willing and able to take the time and the trouble to master the method.

Labor Attendants

In his writings, Read speaks of the supporting people during the labor as being the obstetrician and nurse or nurse–midwife. It is these attendants who guide the woman's use of the method during her labor experience. He also talks of having had many husbands present through the whole of the labor and delivery, taking an active role in helping their wife to relax and breathe and to provide comfort measures between contractions. While Read makes no generalizations about all husbands being present, he is adamant that the totally unprepared man has no place at the birth of his child. His criterion for selecting husbands who can participate is generally to ask: "Can this husband in particular be of service to his wife by being present at her confinement?"[8] When the answer is "Yes," there is no hesitation.

Summary of Read Method

The Read Method of preparation for childbirth is based on the idea that the birth process need not be painful. Through a complex training program involving education, correct breathing, relaxation, and exercises concurrent with breathing, the pregnant woman is taught to look forward to her childbirth

7. *Ibid.*
8. *Ibid.*

experience and the reward of seeing her child born. The burden of the success of the method is on the educator and on the labor attendants:

> If women are not well prepared and if their attendants have not learned the power of anxiety and doubt, these two combine to destroy the natural peace of parturition.
>
> *Grantly Dick-Read, M.D., M.A.*

LAMAZE METHOD—CHILDBIRTH WITHOUT PAIN

In describing childbirth without pain, Lamaze is quite outspoken about his interpretation of the shortcomings of the Read method. While he recognizes and praises the educational aspects of the training, he is most condemning in his attacks on the "half mystical and half rational mixture" which, he claims, ignores the fact that pain does exist and needs definite measures to abolish it.[9] In point of fact, Read was also outspoken about the rapid breathing being taught by French obstetricians and its lack of necessity and harmfulness to the orderly progress of labor.[10]

Childbirth without pain, according to Lamaze, has its foundation in the basic understanding that pain is an entity. The physical and psychological aspects of pain are inseparable. However, pain and uterine contractions are two distinct phenomena that have been linked in the human mind. The Lamaze method of painless childbirth attempts to undramatize labor with all its negative association and to form new conditioned reflexes that will serve to eliminate the pain associated with contractions by using the individual's own nervous system.

What Is Pain?

Lamaze spends a great deal of time talking about the physiology of pain. His fascination with the nervous system and its responses forms the core of his approach to dealing with pain.

> The nervous system however does not only give life to the assembly (the body). The body is already alive by virtue of the sub-

---

9.   Fernand Lamaze, *Painless Childbirth* (Chicago: Henry Regnery, 1970).
10.   Dick-Read, *op. cit.*

stance it is made of. The nervous system does more, it adapts the working of our body to the changes in the environment. This is the main role, and it is specifically for the exchanges between the body and its surroundings that this specialized "relations officer" has been evolved.

Adaptation is the key. All that follows in the Lamaze Method is an attempt to help the body to adapt. Much of the Lamaze Method comes from his understanding of Russian experimentation in reflexology for he believed that all behavior, even that of higher animals, was a result of either inborn reflexes that are automatic responses or conditioned reflexes that are learned.

Because reflexology plays such a large role in the Lamaze Method, it is important to discuss some of the basic concepts, as interpreted by Lamaze.

Lamaze and Reflexology

The nervous system, in its role of mediating between the body and its surroundings, functions at its most basic level is a reception–response mechanism. A specific stimulus gives rise to a specific response. This phenomenon is reflex activity. Some reflexes are inborn, such as blinking when an object approaches the eye or salivating when food is placed in the mouth. These are termed absolute reflexes and are permanent and stable provided the person has an intact central nervous system. Other reflexes are elicited by special conditions in the person's surroundings. Lamaze describes the physiology of conditioned reflex:

1. All stimuli that impinge on our being are transmitted to the brain, be they from our organs or sensory perception, our skin, our muscles, etc., or from the activities of our internal organs, such as the lungs, heart, stomach, etc. They pass up the various nerves and then through the spinal cord to reach the brain.

2. When a stimulus reaches the brain, it fires off a focus of activity, that is, a certain group of nerve cells start to become active. This focus of activity directly stimulates functions in the absolute reflexes; thus the dog salivates when meat is placed in its mouth, or turns its head toward the sound when the bell rings. In each case the focus of activity is a different one: the one belongs to the reflex of salivation, the other to that of orientation. But if two foci of activity are fired off at the same time, and this is repeated many times, a connection becomes established between the two foci. If the repetitions have been frequent enough, a permanent communication results. This link gives rise, within the brain matter, to a channel or

pathway between the two foci in such a way that if one is activated by means of its stimulus (the bell), the other becomes activated too without its stimulus (the meat) being present. One focus then activates the other—this intercommunication between foci of activity is a temporary one artificially induced by prevailing circumstances and makes it possible for the animal to adapt itself to these circumstances. This liaison constitutes a conditioned reflex.

Lamaze goes on to define four additional concepts which he later incorporates into the method:[11]

1. Stereotyped dynamic system: A group of conditioned reflexes working together for a definite purpose. These systems are deemed stereotyped because they always produce the same result in the same sequence, but they are dynamic because they are in a constant state of flux.

2. Reciprocal induction: The process by which the brain is able to contain areas of excitation. Each time a cerebral center becomes excited the area around it becomes modified so that an area of inhibition forms in inverse proportion to the area of excitation.

3. Signalizing activities of the hemispheres: The property of the hemispheres of the brain to engender conditioned reflexes is called their signalizing activity. Speech as a form of communication serves as a second form of signalization using symbols as the stimulus.

4. Interoception: The internal signalization to the brain from body organs.

Pain in Labor

If, as Lamaze contends, pain in labor is a conditioned response, then it follows that people can be conditioned to have painless labors as well. Russian researcher Vekvolvosky indicated that a combination of high emotions and conditioned reflexes combined to interfere with contractions which became painful as a result.[12] Culturally accepted beliefs are imprinted and serve as a secondary signal. Fear of pain predisposes the woman to heightened sensation. Fear of pain is not alone as a predisposing factor, according to Lamaze. Fear of complications, even death, play a part. Unfortunate social circumstances surrounding the pregnancy or birth of this child,

11.   Lamaze, op. cit., p. 45.
12.   I. Velvovsky, et al., Painless Childbirth through Psychoprophylaxis, trans. David A. Myshne (Moscow: Foreign Languages Publishing House, 1960).

which cause the mother to worry, will also affect her perceptions during labor. But by far the most fear-inducing factor is lack of knowledge. Lamaze recognizes that most women have only a scanty knowledge of conception and pregnancy and of their physiology, and no knowledge about the childbirth process. Those who have gained some knowledge have often obtained it from poor sources such as relatives who have themselves had poor experiences or from literature that has dramatized the delivery process to make more emotional reading. Given all these pain enlargers acting collectively on the woman in labor, it is no wonder that fear of pain alone can wear out the cerebral processes and by so doing exhaust the coping powers of the higher centers. Lamaze used the basic premise that pain in childbirth depends on the functional state of the brain, which is influenced by conditioned reflexes formed by prior education, formal and informal, and by the emotional blows created by words, to serve as the guide for reorganizing the activities of the mind to cope more effectively with labor.

Lamaze and Pain Suppression

Lamaze defines *psychoprophylaxis* as the prevention of pain through the use of words.[13] The method attempts to abolish pain by preventing the occurrence and development of pain through knowledge of pain genesis. In the untrained woman there is the presence of conditioned connections with the pain centers in the brain and no reciprocal inhibition to conteract. The woman trained in the psychoprophylactic method of Lamaze has worked to destroy the obnoxious conditioning as well as to increase reciprocal inhibitions to a level that will successfully hold back painful stimuli. The first is accomplished by education, which removes apprehension, fear, and depression by undramatizing labor, thus destroying distressing associations. The second is accomplished by formation of new conditioned reflexes, namely the contraction–respiration reflex. This reflex is taught during pregnancy as shallow, quick breaths to be begun as soon as the woman is aware of uterine contraction. In actual labor, the uterine contraction becomes a signal for specific respiration rather than pain, that is, the contractions initiate the conditioned reflex that high channels the stimuli from the uterine interoceptors to the center for respiration rather than the pain center. Lamaze calls this focal diversion an analgesic maneuver. He recommends that this positive maneuver be practiced by the woman during the first stage of labor. During the second stage of labor, she will practice controlled expulsion.

13.   Lamaze, *op. cit.*

Lamaze and Breathing Exercises

Lamaze reports three justifications for breathing exercises:[14]

1. Breathing exercises allow the woman to make a conscious appraisal of the anatomical relationship between organs directly or indirectly related to the labor process.
2. Breathing exercises provide physical training for a physical event with the intent of building good muscle tone and controlling the muscles.
3. Breathing exercises provide an oxygen-rich gaseous exchange.

Preparatory Breathing Exercises

The preparatory exercise that is intended to link the theoretical teaching with the physical reality, by allowing the woman to study the anatomical relationships within her own body, is taught with an admonition to analyze carefully the relationships that had been taught.

> DO:
> Take a deep inspiration, through the nose if possible; breathe out, doing the expiration in two stages:
> A. Passive Stage. With an open mouth, let air escape freely from lungs until an equilibrium is reached.
> B. Active Stage. Using abdominal muscles, imagine a candle about two feet away and blow hard enough to bend flame but not to blow it out.
>
> THINK:
> • Inspiration . . . Diaphragm . . . Uterine Fundus . . . Vertical Compression
> • Expiration . . . Abdominal Muscles . . . Collapse of Ribs . . . Lateral Compression of Uterus and Elevation of the Pelvis.

This exercise is practiced three times a day for three to five minutes while lying on a couch on the back. Respirations may be altered from five to nine times per minute.

14. *Ibid.*

Breathing Technique for Labor

The actual breathing technique for use during labor is a shallow quickened breath combined with conscious muscular relaxation, particularly of the abdominal muscles, pelvic floor muscles, and the muscles of the shoulders, back, and buttocks. Because this is a contraction–respiration reflex, it should be carried out from the time the excitation leaves the uterus regardless of the intensity of the contraction. Lamaze does recognize that the shallow and quickened breathing really starts to have effect from the time dilatation reaches the size of a quarter. Muscular relaxation, however, is useful from start to finish of labor with a need to adhere to it in between contractions at about the time of quarter-sized dilatation. In practicing the shallow and quickened breathing, the woman is told to carry out shallow quickened breathing with muscular relaxation six different times a day. Typical instruction might include:

- Lungs should not be too full or too empty
- Breathing can either be through nose or mouth
- Respiration exchange should be equal
- Do not try to breathe too shallowly or too quickly
- Shoulders must not be shrugged
- Practice lying down: flat on back; at times on one side; at times sitting up

Breathing Techniques for Delivery

The breathing technique for use during delivery is based on breath-holding and muscular control. The important things that the woman must know is the right time to push and the right way to push. The right time is when the contraction is at its maximum intensity. The right way is to block air in the lungs, touch the chin to the chest and keep it there by rounding shoulders forward and downward using hands and arms to maintain the position. At the same time the woman tries to relax the pelvic floor. It is incorrect to tell her to bear down as if she is defecating, because that maneuver squeezes the rectum and vagina and in fact can retard the delivery.

Lamaze and Relaxation

Lamaze contends that muscular relaxation is an active phenomenon as far as the brain is concerned, that is, he describes relaxation as occurring when the brain transmits a negative order to a motor organ, motor centers in the brain become extinguished, and the muscle stops working immediately. Therefore, if muscular relaxation is an active phenomenon, it can be actively controlled. Lamaze believes that the woman, by practicing muscular control, learns to recognize the muscles that play a useful part in her childbirth and how to use them efficiently. She also learns to identify the muscles that play no part and are likely to be antagonistic to contractions or the delivery process. By practicing controlled relaxation "from the moment of the first contraction appears," she is able to get the maximum efficiency from her brain in raising her threshold of painful perception by putting into practice all the reflexes she acquired during her preparation.

Relaxation exercises: Practice lying down on the back (later on the side or sitting up)

1. Start with the respiratory exercise—breathe in, breathe out, blow out candle (passive interval serves no purpose), repeat two, three, or four times.
2. Tone up the muscles by contracting them in turn, small groups at a time, strenuously but not with exaggeration.
3. Stop all contractions and stay relaxed.
4. Maintain control over this muscular relaxation.
5. End the exercises with the same respiratory ones as at the start.

During successive practice sessions, progress can be checked by mobilization of different parts of the body. This exercise should be practiced four times a day a maximum of five minutes each time.

Lamaze on Medication

Lamaze states that the psychoprophylactic method is an analgesic maneuver. He implies that obstetrical anesthesia and analgesia are unnecessary when the method is properly applied. "Anesthesia should be used only in cases reckoned by the obstetrician or midwife to be difficult."[15]

Labor Attendants

Among the considerations that Lamaze lists for favorable outcomes are adequate materials and facilities and a receptive staff to support the mother

15. *Ibid.* p. 175.

during labor. It is essential to the experience of the mother that all the staff with whom she come in contact be thoroughly versed in the method. "Everything must create an impression of ease and security. The departurient must not feel the need to fall back on herself or be on the defensive." [16] Further, the woman should be helped right through labor by a qualified person—whom Lamaze identifies as a doctor, midwife, or specially trained nurse.

Summary of Lamaze Method

The Lamaze Method of preparation for childbirth is, like the Read Method, based on the idea that childbirth need not be painful. Unlike the Read, however, this method finds its rationale in the neurophysiology of pain and Russian experimentation with conditioned reflexes. Combining controlled muscular relaxation and breathing techniques, the Lamaze Method offers women the opportunity to participate consciously in the birth of their children.

> The preparation can be offered and should be offered without discrimination to every pregnant woman. As we have already said, this instruction is but a stage in the education that all young girls should be given during adolescence. This is why we feel that its general propagation is absolutely essential to the radical change in the mental outlook that a pregnant woman has towards her confinement, regardless of the method used.
>
> *Fernand Lamaze, M.D.*

THE ECLECTIC APPROACHES

It is doubtful that there is very much pure Read, or pure Lamaze being taught in the United States today. Most of the courses offered in preparation for labor and delivery combine features of both the Read and Lamaze methods. This development has been more a function of evolution than a deliberate attempt to define a third approach. These combined approaches are referred to in this book as eclectic. They incorporate not only Read and Lamaze but also the outstanding contribution of American childbirth education—the husband/

16. *Ibid.* p. 171.

labor coach. Where Read felt that the obstetrician should direct labor, and Lamaze felt that only physicians, midwives, or specially trained nurses were qualified to support the trained woman, American childbirth education has moved in the direction of assisting the interested husband in assuming the role of labor coach to his wife. Unlike the passive support roles expected by the European approaches, the American husband/labor coach has a specific active role during preparation and during the labor process itself.

Recognizing the Biopsychosocial Unit

The eclectic approaches—and there are many, each taking the name of the person who offered the modification that made it different—seem to be better balanced than either the early Read or Lamaze methods. This outcome may be based on an acceptance of the concept that the human being is a biopsychosocial unit. While this statement may sound like jargon, it has meaning, particularly when related back to the theory of adaptation. If one accepts that each person is a composite of his or her biological being, psychological being, and social being all interacting at once, then it follows that any attempt to help a person cope with stressful situations will have to consider the biological, psychological, and social factors involved. So it is with childbirth education which is, after all, an attempt to provide means whereby people can cope with a stressful situation. The eclectic approaches offer the biological techniques (structural and physiological) developed by Lamaze with the psychological support of the teachings of Read and the social reinforcement of the husband/labor coach, and the childbirth team.

Pain and the Eclectics

Many believe that it is unreasonable for women to expect pain-free labors no matter how well trained they are. However, it is possible to alter pain perception appreciably using Lamaze techniques, probably for exactly the reasons that Lamaze has described, namely reciprocal inhibition. In addition, correct factual information about the labor process and the surroundings in which it will take place serve as a psychoanalgesia by eliminating a large amount of the fear that results in unnecessary tension and increased pain. If pain is reduced to manageable proportions the average women can deal effectively with what she perceives, providing she receives encouragement and support from the people around her during her labor.

PHYSICAL PREPARATION

All the preparation that the expectant mother receives merges in her mind to create a whole that enables her to perform with confidence. The entire preparation could therefore be said to be psychological preparation. But for purposes of aligning the training with the biopsychosocial model, it will be discussed as physical training, psychological preparation, and social preparation. The physical preparation falls into two categories. Those activities intended to prepare the body to undergo the stress of labor and delivery, and those self-help tools that can be used during labor.

Preparing the Body

Body mechanics

The first step in preparing the body for physical activities is to be sure it is in good alignment. All too often, the pregnant woman stands with poor posture. If she can be helped to stand correctly, it will not only improve the alignment of her pelvic area, but it will also help her to improve her ability to ventilate the lungs (Fig. 3-7).

After posture, the next area of physical preparation is physical fitness for labor. Because it is impossible to turn a sedentary woman into an athletically fit woman in the last few weeks of pregnancy, the next best thing is to concentrate on the strengthening of those muscles that will be used most during labor or delivery. There is no magical set of exercises that is substantially better and safer than any other set of exercises for a pregnant woman to do. The exercises offered by Read are just as effective as the ones below (Figs. 3-8 through 3-11).

An alternative exercise for the woman who does not feel muscle activity with the tailor press is the tailor stretch (Fig. 3-10). The woman sits with her legs out in front, slightly part, her feet rotated outward. She raises her arms straight up on a level with her shoulders (parallel to the floor). She breathes in. As she lets her breath out, she leans forward, keeping her back straight and arms parallel to the floor. If the exercise is done correctly, one feels a strong stretching along the backs of the legs.

Positioning for Comfort

This aspect of physical preparation is helpful not only for labor but also for the remainder of the pregnancy. It is a simple thing to use pillows and

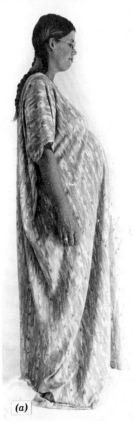 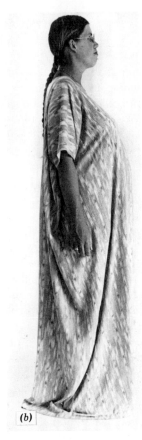

Figure 3–7.

(a) Poor body alignment leads to back problems. (b) Good posture—head and shoulders back, spine in alignment.

positioning to make the pregnant woman comfortable so that she can get adequate rest and sleep (Fig. 3–12). Yet many women resort to all kinds of attempts to get comfortable including trying to sleep sitting in a chair because they find it so difficult to be comfortable until someone shows them how.

Caution! Many women find that they cannot lie on their back at all in the latter part of pregnancy because of the "vena cava syndrome" brought about by the weight of the baby on the inferior vena cava. For these women, side lying only is recommended.

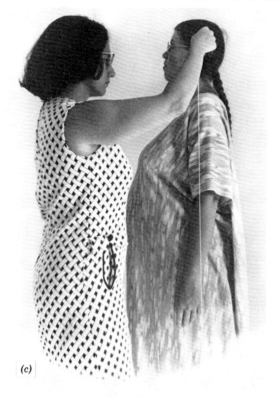

(c)

Figure 3-7. (continued)

(c) The childbirth educator can demonstrate the mother's postural alignment by holding a weighted string at about ear height. If posture is good, string will fall approximately in line with shoulders, waist, hips, and knees. (Used with permission.)

SELF-HELP TOOLS

Probably the most publicized part of the entire preparation for childbirth is the series of relaxation and breathing techniques which are taught as self-help tools that the mother can use during labor. Partly based on the Read theory that if the woman can relax, her own body will not impede the progress of labor, and partly on the Lamaze conception that creating an alternative focus of cerebral activity will alter pain perception, the relaxation and breathing techniques serve to aid the woman in coping with her contractions.

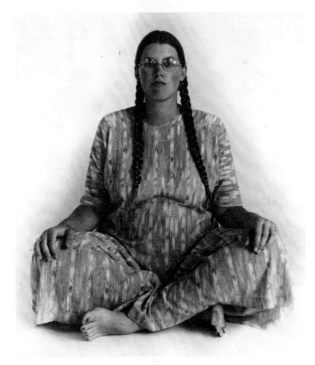

Figure 3–8.

Tailor sitting—releases strain on low back muscles. (Used with permission.)

Conscious Relaxation

Conscious relaxation is precisely what the name implies. It is a deliberate attempt to relax all the body that is not needed to accomplish a particular activity. For the woman in labor, that activity is the contracting of the uterus. By consciously relaxing all nonworking muscles, the woman is able to conserve her energy and at the same time not use up available circulating oxygen unnecessarily. Because most people in our civilized society are somewhat tense all the time, it is necessary for the woman to learn how to relax. In the family-centered approach to preparation for childbearing, learning how to relax also serves as the beginning of the teamwork between father and mother which will be carried out during actual labor. The mother's role is to master the skill of relaxing. The father's role is to recognize signs of tension, call them to the mother's attention, and help her to relax more effectively (Figs. 3–13, 3–14). This is accomplished during the training period, which

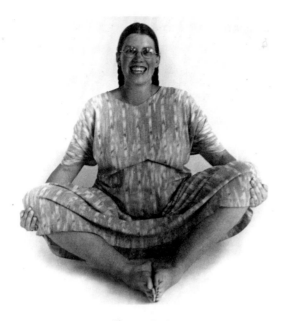

Figure 3–9.

Tailor press—to avoid jerking low back muscles, be sure that mother places hands under knees, pulling up with hands while pressing down with knees. (Used with permission.)

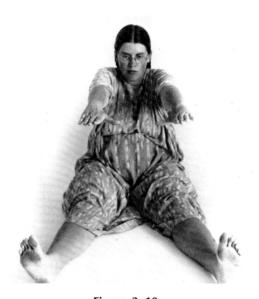

Figure 3–10.

Tailor stretch—done with straight back and outstretched arms parallel to floor. Fingers do *not* reach for toes. (Used with permission.)

51

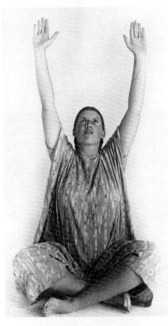

Figure 3–11.

Tailor reach—stretching up to grasp an imaginary bar, just beyond the fingertips. (Used with permission.)

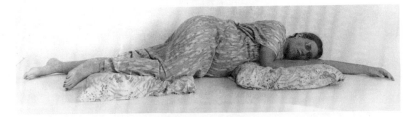

Figure 3–12.

Side lying becomes very important to avoid "vena cava syndrome." Positioning with pillows helps. (Used with permission.)

should probably extend for about the last six weeks to two months of pregnancy. Practice during the training period is done by the couple at their own convenience (Figs. 3–15, 3–16). And, since controlled relaxation is the key to coping with labor contractions, the better trained the couple, the more likely they will have the kind of experience they would like to have.

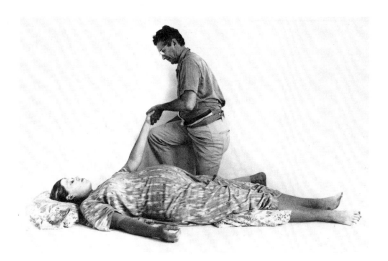

Figure 3–13.

The best way for the coach to check the arm for relaxation is to grasp the hand as though shaking hands and lift. The arm should feel heavy and swing freely from the shoulder. (Used with permission.)

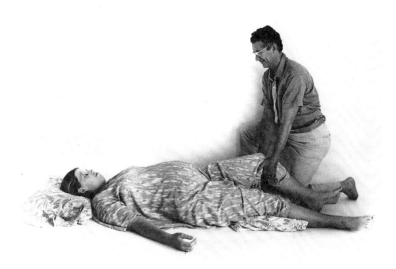

Figure 3–14.

When checking the leg for relaxation, the coach can avoid tickling by placing both hands behind the knee and lifting. The relaxed foot should slide along the floor. (Used with permission.)

Figure 3-15. (*a*)
CONTROLLED RELAXATION—PRELIMINARY ROUTINE.

Husband's cues	Wife's reactions	What to look for
1. "Stretch legs down"	Push down through legs; keeping foot flexed, push heel as far as possible	Tight muscles the length of the leg; foot held tightly
"Relax"	Let legs flop	Contrast loose muscles with those tense during exercise
2. "Stretch spine"	Pull top of spine up while pushing the lower portion down	Tension throughout torso, will probably include shoulders and possibly arms and legs
"Relax"	Let spine fall back against pillows	Body loses tension; note how she looks when relaxed
3. "Contract buttocks"	Tighten the muscles of the buttocks	Body will be slightly raised in the area of the lower back as tight buttocks create a bridge
"Relax"	Let all muscles go allowing back to fall back on pillows	Back will rest on support—no space visible under lower spine
4. "Stretch arms"	Push down through arms, through palms of hands; extend fingers reaching as far as possible without lifting shoulders	Tension along arms, and in shoulders; fingers tense
"Relax"	Allow arms to flop	Arms resting loosely at side; fingers slightly curled in repose
5. "Shrug shoulders"	Bring shoulders as high as possible beside head without lifting them off pillows	Shoulders tense, neck may be able to see blood vessels standing out; head held rigidly
"Relax"	Let shoulders flop back to normal	All parts rest against support
6. "Frown"	Make a face and hold as tightly as possible	Facial muscles taut; worried look; head rigid; neck tense
"Relax"	Let your face return to normal	Face in repose; head resting on pillow

Figure 3-15. (*b*)
CONTROLLED RELAXATION PRACTICE.

Husband's cues	Wife's reactions	What to look for
1. "Contract right arm"	Make a fist of right hand and raise a few inches	Check to see if wife has eyes focused; check left arm and both legs; give direction to relax
"Relax"	Arm should drop back on support	Check to see that arm drops and is not consciously lowered
2. "Contract left arm"	Same as for right arm	Same as for right arm
"Relax"		
3. "Contract left leg"	Pull toes of foot as close to body as possible (flex foot); tighten muscles of leg as if it were to be raised	Check for eye focus; check both arms and right leg—it is especially difficult in the beginning to tense one leg and relax the other; check to see if buttocks are tense (hard)
"Relax"	Leg should go limp	Check leg for relaxation before going on
4. "Contract both arms"	Tighten both fists	Check for tension in neck and face; check legs
"Relax"	Both arms should drop	Same as with one arm; both should drop and not be lowered
5. "Contract both legs"	Flex both feet	Check both arms and head and neck for tension
"Relax"	Both legs should go limp	Check legs for relaxation
6. "Contract both shoulders"	Shrug shoulders	Check hands and both legs; observe face for tension
"Relax"	Let shoulders return to normal position	Check neck for tension

Reprinted with permission from Sasmor, JL: *What Every Husband Should Know About Having a Baby.* Chicago, Nelson-Hall, 1972.

Learning to relax consciously is an activity that always sounds easier than it is. One way for people to become aware of tension and relaxation is to begin with a progressive muscular relaxation exercise. Once learned, it is also an excellent means of bringing relaxation to a tense body so that the person can fall asleep.

In teaching couples, it is not a bad idea to have the fathers try to do the progressive relaxation before the mothers. This sequence lets them feel tension and relaxation and helps them appreciate the effort that their partners have to make to relax consciously.

Selective Muscular Relaxation

Controlled relaxation of selected groups of muscles is the primary self-help tool. Because the labor stimulus, the contracting uterus, is not active for the practice session, other muscles groups are used. It should be clearly indicated that these simulated contractions will not be used during labor when the uterus itself is active. However, for practice purposes, the woman will be asked to contract the muscles in a specific part of her body, while deliberately trying to relax all other muscle groups. During this time, the father should be taught how to check for relaxation or if he finds tension, how to assist his partner in relaxing the tense muscles groups. For some women this assistance will be by means of verbal cues such as "Release your right arm." For others, the cue will be a tactile one such as stroking the tense part (Fig. 3–15).

Training to master relaxation is a psychomotor skill that responds best to brief, regularly scheduled practice sessions rather than long, irregularly scheduled ones.

BREATHING TECHNIQUES

The breathing techniques that are taught cannot stand alone without controlled relaxation. They are always executed with the conscious attempt to relax all parts of the body not actively involved in the current effort. Because they require effort themselves, the breathing techniques should be used only as they are needed.

Breathing Basics

All breathing techniques have four basic components. The first is that as the start of each contraction is perceived, the woman picks an immovable spot and focuses her eyes. This action focuses her attention on responding to her sensations. Second, she takes a deep breath. As she exhales, she attempts consciously to relax her whole body. This deep breath is a clue to her coach that she is perceiving another contraction. Third, she carries out all the breathing techniques as chest breathing, attempting to keep the abdominal muscles relaxed. Fourth, at the end of the contraction, she takes in one or more deep breaths to help restore the oxygen balance, which may have been disturbed during the contraction.

Although many personal variations have appeared and been taught, only three primary breathing techniques exist for use during labor. If these are learned and learned well, any variation can be added without detracting from the techniques, provided there is a sound basis for the variation. The three techniques are: slow chest breathing, shallow breathing, and pant-blow breathing. It was fashionable at one time to link the techniques with the phases of the first stage of labor. However, if they are to be truly self-help tools, they should be available at the discretion and need of the woman rather than according to the labels that have been given them.

Slow Rhythmic Breathing

This slow relaxing breathing is taught as a chest-breathing technique. It is executed by inhaling through the nose and exhaling slowly through pursed lips. The rhythm is maintained by breathing between six and nine times per minute of practice contraction. Each practice contraction is begun by a deep breath and ended by a deep breath. These deep breaths are not included in the six to nine count.

Because this technique is the easiest to do and provides the best exchange of oxygen, it should be used as long as it is effective in controlling the perception of the pain related to uterine contractions. When it is no longer effective, an additional behavior is added. This behavior is called *effleurage* and is a light abdominal massage (Figs. 3–16, 3–17). It is coordinated with the breathing technique, thus increasing the concentration necessary to carry it out, and thereby interfering with pain perception. Effleurage is done with relaxed arms and hands, with just the fingertips touching the skin of the abdomen. The woman follows the outline of her uterus starting at the pubis symphysis, moving her fingertips up around the outside of the uterus and

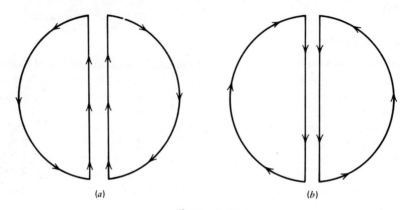

(a)   (b)

Figure 3–16.

(a) Effleurage is a light fingertip massage beginning with both hands held loosely at the symphysis pubis and slowly raising with the inhaled breath. As the woman exhales, her hands slowly follow the outer contours of her abdomen. (b) Effleurage variation. Some women prefer to start at the symphysis pubis and follow the outer contour of the abdomen, raising their hands while inhaling, returning down the inner aspect while exhaling. This may be related to handedness.

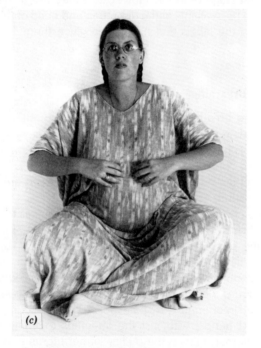

Figure 3–16. (c)

Effleurage—gentle abdominal massage in conjunction with relaxation and breathing techniques.

58

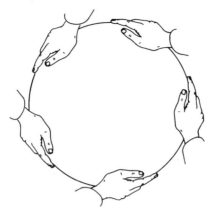

Figure 3–17.

Sometimes the woman prefers the coach to do the effleurage for her. With a slightly cupped hand, using only the fingertips, the coach starts at the upper outer aspect of the abdomen on the opposite side and gently draws his hand down, across, and up. Take starting position and begin again.

then returning to starting position. As she raises her hands, she breathes in and, as she lowers her hands, she breathes out (Fig. 3–2).

Shallow Breathing

Shallow breathing is a technique for use later in labor. It is intended to reduce the intraabdominal pressure created when the diaphragm is lowered with deep breathing. When one is doing shallow breathing correctly, the diaphragm will flutter, particularly important at the peak of the contraction. Shallow breathing is a variable technique, as it is executed by the woman in exact response to what she perceives her contraction to be. She starts by taking a deep breath, then immediately switches to breathing in and out through her mouth lightly and quickly. If she could hear the sound she is making, it would sound like "heh." If she is making puffing sounds that sound like "huh," she is breathing too deeply in the chest. As soon as she switches to the shallow breathing, she should also place the tip of her tongue behind her upper front teeth and smile slightly which will help reduce the mouth dryness caused by evaporation (Fig. 3–18). Because the contraction will follow a curve with a beginning, a peak, and an end, the breathing technique will also follow a curve of activity, slowly building up to a peak, remaining at the peak for a period of time, and then returning to a more normal pace. As at the

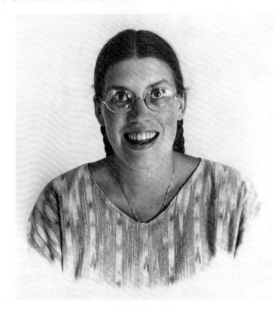

Figure 3–18.

To reduce mouth dryness while practicing shallow breathing, the tongue should be placed behind the upper front teeth and the woman should smile slightly. (Used with permission.)

beginning, the contraction ends with a deep breath. If it has been a difficult contraction, several deep breaths will help to restore the oxygen balance, which may be disturbed by prolonged difficult contractions.

When shallow breathing by itself is no longer effective in controlling pain perception, effleurage can be added. To coordinate effleurage with shallow breathing the woman must imagine that her abdomen is divided into quarter sections. With every four respiratory exchanges she will move the distance of one quarter of effleurage (Fig. 3–19).

Transition Breathing

During transition, it is necessary for the women to have a very rhythmical pattern to follow. Concentration becomes difficult and the internal pressures are almost uncontrollable. This is the time when she will feel the urge to push her baby out, but the cervix is not yet ready. Therefore, with the urge to push

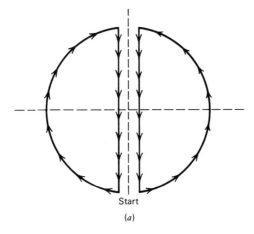

Start

(a)

Figure 3–19. (a)

When doing effleurage to accompany the shallow breathing, the mental image to convey is that the abdomen is divided into four quarters. For every four breaths, the hands move smoothly through one quarter.

she must work to counteract the sensation by interfering with the pushing mechanism.

Human anatomy dictates that we bear down by filling the lungs and using the thoracic and abdominal muscles. In transition, the woman has to blow air out of her lungs and try to keep her abdominal muscles relaxed.

Therefore, transition breathing is a pattern of rhythmic shallow breathing alternating with short staccato blowing, reverting to repeated blowing out with the urge to push. An easy pattern to learn is six breaths and a blow. Like all the breathing techniques it begins and ends with a deep breath. When practicing, the woman should have someone else call out the urge to push because it occurs in labor without her volition and she needs to be able to respond automatically.

Expulsion

Expulsion does not require a breathing technique so much as the ability to hold the breath and get into the best position to push. Because it is effective to push only at the peak of a contraction, the woman should let the contraction build by taking in a deep breath, letting it out, taking in another, letting it out,

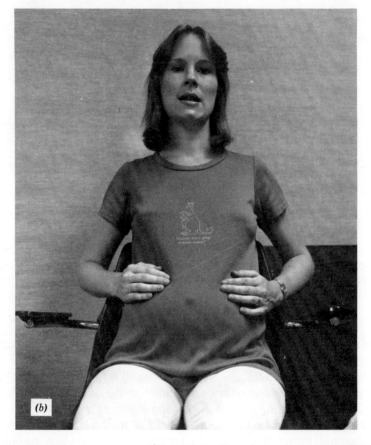

Figure 3–19. (*b*)

Practicing shallow breathing with effleurage. (Used with permission.)

taking in a third full deep breath, and holding it. Then she should get into effective pushing position by rounding her shoulders, lowering her chin on her chest, grasping her legs behind the knees, and leaning down with all her muscles onto the contraction (Fig. 3–20).

Between contractions, it is recommended that the woman rest and do slow rhythmic breathing to restore oxygen and conserve energy. In the delivery room, the only difference in executing the expulsion technique is that the hands will be on a hand-hold rather than behind the knees. But the breathing pattern and position are essentially the same.

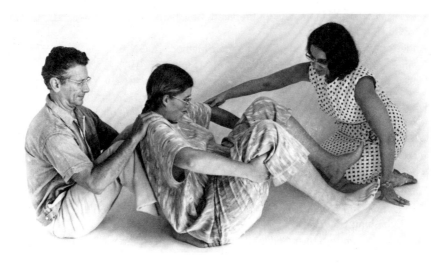

Figure 3–20.

It is possible to simulate the position for labor room pushing by having the coach use his flexed legs as the back support. (Used with permission.)

SUMMARY

Self-help approaches to childbirth have developed over the past three decades. Today's parents benefit from the theory of Dr. Grantly Dick-Read and the techniques and practices of Dr. Fernand Lamaze. Modifications have developed over the years and represent evolution rather than rapid changes in practice.

BIBLIOGRAPHY

———— Childbirth by the Lamaze Method. *Mothers-to-be*, Fall, 1970.
———— *Comfort During Pregnancy.* New York, Maternity Center Assn.
———— *Preparation for Childbearing.* New York, Maternity Center Assn.
———— *Relaxation and Breathing.* New York, Maternity Center Assn.

————"Whatever Happened to Prepared Childbirth—Readers Respond," *JOGN* **4**:3, May/June 1975.

Anderson J: A Clarification of the Lamaze Method. *JOGN* **6**:2, Mar/Apr 1977.

Bean C: *Methods of Childbirth*. New York: Doubleday, 1972.

Bing ED: *Six Practical Lessons for An Easier Childbirth* (New York: Grosset and Dunlap, 1967).

Bonstein I: *Psychoprophylactic Preparation for Painless Childbirth*. London, Morrison & Gibb, Ltd, 1958.

Bradley R: *Husband-Coached Childbirth*. New York, Harper & Row, 1965.

Buxton CL: *A Study of Psychophysical Methods for Relief of Pain in Childbirth*. Philadelphia, W. B. Saunders, 1962.

Chabon I: *Awake and Aware*. New York: Delacorte Press, 1966.

Ewy D, Ewy R: *Preparation for Childbirth—A Lamaze Guide*. Boulder, Colo, Pruett Publishing Co, 1970.

Hazell L: *Common Sense Childbirth*. New York, G. P. Putnam & Sons, 1969.

Jacobson E: *How to Relax and Have Your Baby*. New York, McGraw-Hill, 1965.

Karmel M: *Thank You, Dr. Lamaze*. Philadelphia, J. B. Lippincott, 1959.

Kitzinger S: *The Experience of Birth*. London, Keplinger Publishing Co, 1974.

———— *An Approach to Antenatal Teaching*. London, National Childbirth Trust, 1968.

———— *The Experience of Childbirth*. New York, Taplinger, 1972.

Joseph S: Whatever Happened to Prepared Childbirth? *JOGN* **5**:1, Jan/Feb 1976.

Sasmor JL: *What Every Husband Should Know About Having a Baby*. Chicago: Nelson-Hall Co., 1972.

Scott JR, Rose NB: Effect of Psychoprophylaxis on Labor and Delivery in Primiparas. *New England Journal of Medicine*, May 27, 1976.

Wessell H, Ellis HF (eds): *The Practice of Natural Childbirth*, 45th ed. New York, Harper & Row, 1972.

Wright E: *The New Childbirth*. New York: Hart Publishing Co., 1966.

PART TWO

STRATEGIES FOR TEACHING CHILDBIRTH EDUCATION: A NURSING PROCESS APPROACH

Within the past decade, the definition of current nursing practice has emerged with greater clarity than at any time since the writings of Florence Nightingale. No longer viewed as a static entity, nursing as a process is dynamic, responding to the changes in society's health care needs and the evolving health care system. The basis of nursing process is the scientific method, or problem-solving approach, which is a constant interchange between intellectual skills and actual physical activities for the purpose of testing ideas in the real world. This same interplay is apparent in the four steps of the nursing process: assessment, planning, implementation, and evaluation. Central to all activities is the client and the nurse–client relationship.

Childbirth education is an integral part of nursing practice. As such, childbirth education can and should be considered in terms of the nursing process.

The assessment phase of the nursing process is the focus of Chapter 4. Consideration is given to the client concept and how that concept will influence the assessment perspective from the individual to the family to the community. Data collection and analysis related to childbirth education are reviewed.

65

Chapter 5 deals with planning for childbirth education, according to it all of the respect and careful consideration due any quality educational venture. The chapter progresses from philosophical development to objective writing to teaching strategy selection.

The topics presented in Chapter 6 are related to the implementation of childbirth education programs but reflect the revolution in nursing practice that has occurred in the 1970s. Professional nurses are now held accountable for nursing decisions. State Nurse Practice Acts have expanded the definition of nursing; but with new privileges comes greater responsibility. Nurses in many states now have freedom to choose how they will practice and must carefully consider all of the ramifications of private practice. Adequate preparation, obtaining credentials, and payment for services are but three of many issues yet to be resolved.

The final chapter in this part, Chapter 7, deals with the subject of evaluation. This chapter presents evaluation as an integral continuation of the nursing process rather than a goal. Educational evaluation is comparable to any evaluation, although it is often misused. Evaluation, as presented in this chapter, merely represents the relationship of actual behavior to predetermined criteria. A variety of suggestions is offered for the collection of data on learner behavior and teacher behavior.

The information in this part is designed for the nurse who is involved in the planning or development of a childbirth education program. Rather than giving a cookbook approach which dictates specific activities, it provides the professional nurse with issues and approaches that can be taken into consideration and adapted or modified in response to the particular demands of each individual situation.

Chapter 4

Childbirth Education, Nursing Process, and Assessment

Strategies for teaching childbirth education are no less important than teaching strategies in other educational fields. However, historically, the major emphasis in education for childbearing has been on a method of preparation or content. This emphasis has often left the quality of the educational experience wanting. In order to widen the scope of understanding, consideration should be given to the teaching–learning process, of which content is only a part, and the nursing process, which serves as a framework for developing childbirth education experiences.

TEACHING–LEARNING PROCESS

Teaching is an interpersonal process. It involves an interaction between a teacher and at least one learner. Learning is an intrapersonal process. It involves the gaining of some knowledge or skill that results in some change in behavior. The overall teaching–learning process is an integrated, multiphasic problem-solving process. It involves assessing, planning, implementing, and evaluating both long- and short-term goals. Understanding this process has far-reaching implications for developing relevant, high-quality childbirth education programs that will retain their quality over time.

67

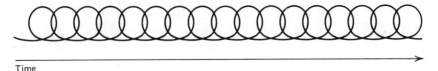

Time

Figure 4–1.

Problem-solving incidents over a period of time.

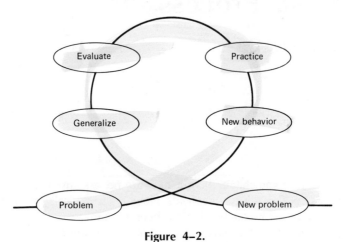

Figure 4–2.

A problem-solving loop.

Miles's Model

Mathew Miles developed a model for looking at group processes that adapts
very easily to almost any attempt to visualize problem-solving processes, of
which the nursing process and educational process are but two.[1] The first
concept to be understood is that a process occurs at a point in time and over a
period of time (Fig. 4–1). Therefore, in Miles's model the process is dia-
grammed as a spiral continuum, each loop representing a problem-solving
episode (Fig. 4–2) and all of the loops connected representing the process
(Fig. 4–1). If this continuity can be conceptualized, it is easy to understand the
nature of the process.

Because the teaching–learning process involves both parties of the interaction, at any point in time there will be two episode loops in operation, one

1.   Matthew Miles, *Learning to Work in Groups: A Program Guide for Educational Leaders*
(New York: Bureau of Publications, Teachers College, Columbia University, 1959).

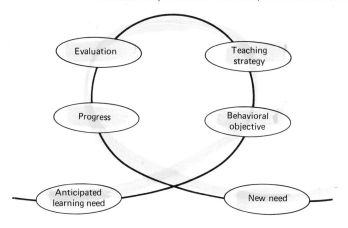

Figure 4–3.

A problem-solving loop from the teacher's perspective.

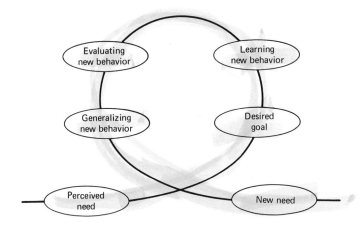

Figure 4–4.

A problem-solving loop from the learner's perspective.

superimposed on the other. One episode represents the problem-solving that the teacher uses (Fig. 4–3); the other represents the problem-solving used by the learner to meet his needs (Fig. 4–4).

When these two loops function concurrently, in harmony, then learning will take place. If either loop is broken or eliminated, learning will definitely be hindered.

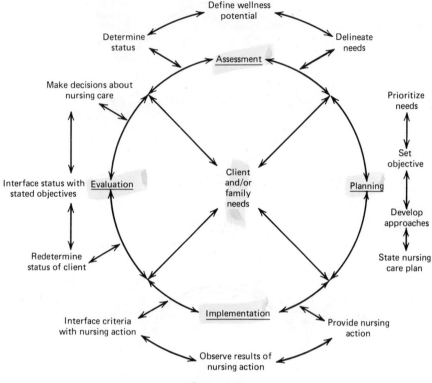

Figure 4–5.

University of South Florida Nursing Process Model.

NURSING PROCESS MODEL

In 1974, the faculty of the College of Nursing of the University of South Florida refined a model for understanding the nursing process as it was expressed in the literature.[2] In an attempt to provide a detailed guide that all practicing nurses could use to apply the nursing process, they recognized that professional nurses operate from individual frames of references that represent personal beliefs, values commitment, and points of view that are culturally developed. However, given that individual nurses will apply the model within their own frame of reference, the nursing process model is offered as Fig. 4–5.

2. College of Nursing Faculty, *Nursing Process Model* (Tampa: College of Nursing, University of South Florida, 1974).

Nursing Process Model and Childbirth Education

Direct application of the nursing process model to the practice of childbirth education is a logical step if one accepts that childbirth education is a natural extension of the patient education component of nursing practice. As a part of nursing practice, childbirth education has the right to the same high-quality service as do all areas of direct patient care. Nursing process allows for high-quality, individualized client-centered care.

The Client Concept

The client concept is basic to childbirth education. The concept of client is synonymous with the concept of consumer (of professional services). Unlike the concept of patient, which restricts the consumer to the sick person, that of client offers a broad opportunity for service. The client might be an individual expectant parent, an expectant or new family, or a community seeking to develop a childbirth education program, depending on the services used (Fig. 4–6). Whichever one the client may be, the application of the nursing process model remains the same.

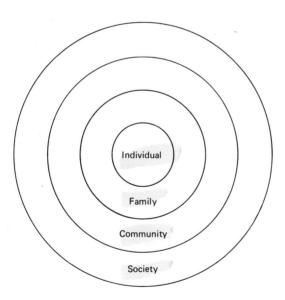

Figure 4–6.

The client concept. A client can be an individual, a family, a community, or society.

Figure 4–7.

Using theoretical frameworks in assessing.

Process model (activity)	Individual client	Family client	Community client
Determine Status	Biopsychosocial assessment	Smilkstein concepts	Grounded theory
Define wellness potential	Dunn's levels of wellness	Smilkstein's model of family functioning: SCEEM	Given reality data, identify assets and liabilities
Delineate needs	From the above data, state client needs—those that can be met by the childbirth educator and those requiring referral		

NURSING PROCESS AND CLIENT ASSESSMENT: THEORETICAL FRAMEWORK

The first phase of the nursing process model (Fig. 4–7) is assessment. Assessment is the process of gathering data from valid and reliable sources for the purpose of identifying client needs. Implied in this definition is the process of data analysis. Needs, Kron says, are concerned with the processes necessary for life and with the person's response to the environment. Concerns, she goes on, are the client's perceptions of his needs or problems. Problems occur when there is a conflict between one or more needs.[3]

The manner in which the nursing process model is applied to a given situation is determined by the theoretical framework that the nurse chooses to apply. There is no right or wrong theoretical base, although some theories seem to have greater scientific relevance than others to given situations.

Determining Individual Status

Individual client assessment includes gathering information about the biological, psychological, and social status of that individual. One helpful way to look at that information is to use the hierarchy of human motivational behav-

3. Thora Kron, *The Management of Patient Care: Putting Leadership Skills to Work,* 4th ed. (Philadelphia: W. B. Saunders, 1976), p. 14.

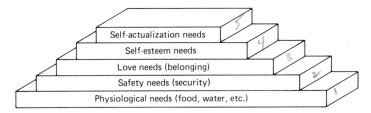

Figure 4–8.

Maslow's Hierarchy of Needs.

ior developed by Dr. Abraham Maslow.[4] Maslow determined that people usually act in a predictable manner based on which order of their personal needs were met, with the understanding that until the primary level of needs were met, the higher levels would be left unmet by the person. The order that he described is shown in Figure 4–8.

During pregnancy, the concerns and problems of the person change as the process of pregnancy continues. The person functions as a biopsychosocial entity, and as such must have consideration given to the variations that are occurring on all three planes as a result of the pregnancy condition. This statement means that in addition to the professional awareness of the client's altered biological state, attention should be given to the client's psychological and social behavior as indicators of her ability to adapt to parenthood (Fig. 4–9).[5]

The childbirth educator is in a unique position to carry out ongoing assessment. Spending an allotted time on a weekly basis provides ample opportunity to gather data through observation and interview. The kinds of data sought would be related to the then current stage of the client's pregnancy. But the elements are applied throughout from the biopsychosocial whole model (Fig. 4–10).

By collecting and analyzing data about the client, the childbirth educator can identify real needs or problems or unusual concerns and assist the client in coping with them or at least will be able to refer her to a more appropriate resource, usually the obstetrician.

4. Abraham Maslow, *Motivation and Personality* (New York: Harper & Row, 1954), pp. 80–106.
5. This model (Fig. 4–9) of the biopsychosocial unit was developed by the author to present the subject of "Sexuality and Pregnancy" to the Sex and Marriage Therapy Conference, Siesta Key, May 1976.

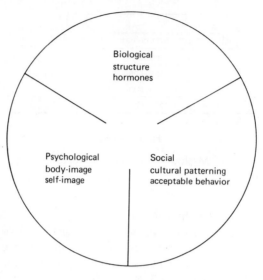

Figure 4–9.

A biopsychosocial model. Note that the space within the model is open in the center. All three planes are constantly interacting with the others to make a total human being.

Determining Family Status

Families, just like individuals, pass through a predictable cycle. The childbirth educator is primarily interested in the family while it is still in the part of the cycle concerned with growth and expansion (Fig. 4–11).[6]

One way of assessing family functioning is described by family physician Gabriel Smilkstein.[7] Smilkstein accepts Hill's taxonomy of family crisis which recognizes the addition of a member as a normative crisis, that is one that is expected. He further defines crisis as any "emotionally or physically significant episode that produces change in the lives of family members." Out of his understanding of the functioning of the family, Smilkstein developed a model of the family in health (Fig. 4–12), which he defines as a nurturing unit that demonstrates functional integrity of five components: commitment, adaptability, mutuality, differentiation, and intimacy.

6. This model (Fig. 4–11) was developed by the author to present family life cycle from a health perspective to medical students at the College of Medicine, University of South Florida, July 1976.
7. Gabriel Smilkstein, "The Family in Trouble—How to Tell," *Journal of Family Practice,* January 1975, pp. 19–24.

Figure 4-10.

Applying a biopsychosocial model to understanding pregnancy.

	First trimester	Second trimester	Third trimester
Biological Assessment			
Structural changes	Signs of pregnancy	Growth of uterus	Growth to term
Hormonal influence	Symptoms of pregnancy	Peaceful period	Letdown, signs of impending labor
Psychological Assessment			
Body-image	Unchanged	"Little mother"	Clumsy, unattractive, unfeminine
Self-image	Ambivalence, rejection, guilt	Acceptance, taking on	Introverted, self-centered
Social Assessment			
Cultural patterning	Variable	Variable	Variable
Acceptable behavior	Happy, excited	"Pregnant woman"	Withdrawn from society

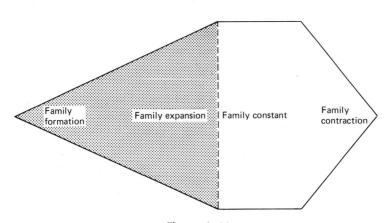

Figure 4-11.

A model for looking at family life cycle.

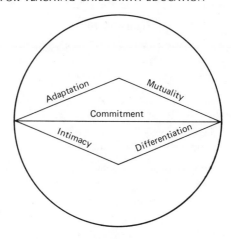

Figure 4–12.

Smilkstein's Model of a Family in Health. *Commitment* is the pledge to be responsible to and for other members of the family. *Adaptation* is the capability for behavior modification in times of crisis or stress. *Mutuality* is the sharing of nurturing needs by family members. *Differentiation* is the measure of individual maturation and development that is allowed within the family structure. *Intimacy* is the caring or loving relationship that exists among family members.

Pregnancy and childbirth are a time of changing family status. The transition can be smooth for some families; for others it is a time of crisis that can be violent enough to precipitate family breakdown.

The role of the childbirth educator is to use the knowledge of family dynamics to identify families at risk. Families at risk have become dysfunctional for some reason. Evidence of family dysfunction, that is the loss of the ability to nurture its members, is the disturbance of one or more of the characteristics identified by Smilkstein. Whether gained through observation or interview, this information would be useful to the other professional members of the childbirth team. First, it allows for the preparation of additional support for the couple during their labor, delivery, and postpartum experience. Second, this information might point to the need for additional professional follow-up after the parents and baby return home. If this information is identified early before the added stress of new responsibilities, it is conceivable that a strong support system for the parents could be established so that they will be in a better position with their new lives.

Determining Community Status

One way of finding out what your community members want is to ask them. Asking can be done indirectly by carrying out interviews with local obstetricians and family doctors who regularly deliver babies as well as with personnel staffing prenatal clinics. Or, asking can be done directly by contacting expectant parents and asking them what they would like. As it is not always easy to have access to the expectant parents individually, it is often possible to reach them through mass media. This approach is especially useful in a small community where the local newspaper is truly community-centered. The family editor or editor of the woman's page is an excellent resource person whose area of interest includes parents. These editors will often run stories about new approaches to expectant parents' education. You can try to elicit their cooperation in getting expectant parents to answer your questions because the answers themselves will tell them more about their readers.

Another approach to discovering, and perhaps even exciting, community interest is to organize a public film showing. A film such as "First Breath,"[8] which not only shows an actual delivery but also provides the audience with a rationale for prepared childbirth from the point of view of an obstetrician, a pediatrician, a psychiatrist, a childbirth educator, and parents themselves, is an excellent medium for attracting those in the community who are already interested and for informing those in the community who would like to know more. By capitalizing on the audience present at a film showing, you can get your questions answered. While this by no means constitutes a random sampling, it at least gives you a starting point.

In essence this is a form of research that places you right in the middle so that you are able to observe firsthand and draw conclusions about the community needs directly from your observations.

Wellness Potential and Client Needs

Wellness potential is defined in the USF Nursing Process Model Glossary as "the highest level of functioning possible for a client given his strength and limitation."[9] Determining wellness potential, therefore, is a sorting process that sifts through the data collected and categorizes information either as a client strength or a client limitation.

8.   Information about the film "First Breath" may be obtained by contacting Childbirth Education Films Inc. 648 Riverside Road, North Palm Beach, Florida 33408.
9.   College of Nursing Faculty, *op. cit.*

Figure 4–13.

Dunn's Levels of Wellness.

Very Favorable Environment

Low-level wellness in
high-level environment

Protected poor health

High-level wellness in
high-level environment

High-level wellness

Death------------------------------------Health · axis--------------------------------------- Optimum
                                                                                                                                                        level
                                                                                                                                                        wellness

Low-level wellness in
low-level environment

Poor health

High-level wellness in
low-level environment

Emergent high-level wellness

Very Unfavorable Environment

The Individual
Physician Halbert Dunn related wellness potential to the individual's state of
health and the state of his environment.[10] This model (Fig. 4–13) holds true
for the pregnancy as well as other medical conditions, and can serve as a
framework for looking at individual strengths and limitations.

The Family
For determining the wellness potential of a family, Smilkstein's model still
holds.[11] Disturbances in any of the components of the family in health model
would be temporary or permanent limitations. To determine family strengths,

10.   Halbert Dunn, "High-Level Wellness for Man and Society" in Jeannette R. Folta, and Edith
S. Deck, *A Sociological Framework for Patient Care* (New York: John Wiley and Sons, 1966, pp.
213–19.
11.   Smilkstein, *op. cit.* pp. 19–20.

Figure 4–14.

Using SCEEM for assessment.

Resources	Family Strengths	Family Limitations
Social	Balanced social interaction	Social isolation or overcommitment
Cultural	Cultural pride	Cultural conflicts
Economic	Economic stability	Economic depression
Educational	Educational adequacy	Educational handicap or inappropriate training
Medical	Absence of disease	Medical deprivation or major medical–surgical problems

which he calls resources, he uses the assessment acronym SCEEM, which stands for social, economic, educational, and medical resources. Using this interpretation is one way for nurses to estimate a family's potential for wellness (Fig. 4–14).

The Community

Community wellness potential may be more than is needed in developing a childbirth education program, unless the focus is restricted to the potential success of the program. For that determination the kind of information to be gathered and sorted falls into two categories: the population and the resources available.

In looking at the population, one needs answers to the following questions: Who are they? What kind of socioeconomic picture do they present? What aspects of their cultural heritage will influence the way they view the childbearing process? What are their perceived needs for childbirth education?

In looking at the resources, one should consider material, human, and intangible resources. Of the three, the intangible resource is the most important part of the community climate, or readiness is the key to the success for the program. This climate includes both consumer and professional readiness for the program. It is also helpful to have material resources such as places to meet, books for libraries, teaching resources and, of course, the human resources—enough qualified teachers to teach in response to the needs of the community.

SUMMARY

Nursing process is a dynamic problem-solving approach to meeting client needs. It provides a model for understanding the total process of childbirth education as a nursing function. The first phase is client assessment.

Client assessment is the process of gathering data about the client for the purpose of defining the client's potential for wellness and delineating the specific needs of the client at that point in time. The childbirth educator needs to consider the three clients with whom it will be necessary to deal in developing a childbirth education program: the individual, the family, and the community. Childbirth education is more than a classroom educational process, involving knowledge, skills, and attitudinal refocusing. To move into the planning phase, the childbirth educator will need to have data on the needs of the individual relevant to biological, psychological and social status; data on the needs of the family relevant to healthful functioning of the unit; and needs of the community relevant to community awareness and readiness for childbirth education. Once the data have been gathered and analyzed, the direction of the planning is foretold.

BIBLIOGRAPHY

Cahill AS: Dual Purpose Tool for Assessing Maternal Needs and Nursing Care *JOGN* **4**:1, Jan/Feb 1975.

Gillies DA, Allyn IB: *Patient Assessment and Management by the Nurse Practitioner.* Philadelphia, W. B. Saunders, 1976.

Green R: *Human Sexuality: A Health Practitioner's Text.* Baltimore, Williams and Wilkins, 1975.

Gruis M: Beyond Maternity: Postpartum Concerns of Mothers *American Journal of Maternal Child Nursing,* May/June 1977.

Kitzinger S: How to Keep Your Marriage Alive After the Baby Comes *American Baby,* June 1973.

Levine N: A Conceptual Model for Obstetric Nursing *JOGN* **5**:2, Mar/Apr 1976.

Murray R, Zentner J: *Nursing Assessment and Health Promotion Through the Life Span.* Englewood Cliffs, NJ, Prentice-Hall, 1975.

Rae W, Riley HD: Learning How to Be a Better Parent *American Baby,* Jan 1976.

Roberts J: Practices in Pre-Natal Education *JOGN* **5**:3, May/Jun, 1976.

Stern T: Establishing Pre-Natal Classes in Small Community: Overcoming Opposition *JOGN* **4:**5, Sept/Oct 1975.

Sumner G, Fritsch J: Postnatal Parental Concerns: The First Six Weeks of Life *JOGN* **6:**3, May/Jun, 1977.

Warren DI, Warren RB: Six Kinds of Neighborhoods, *Psychology Today* **9:**1, June 1975.

——— A Community Leader's Handbook *Psychology Today* **9:**1, June 1975.

Watson J: Who Attends Prepared Childbirth Classes? A Demographic Study of Classes in Rhode Island *JOGN* **6:**2, Mar/Apr 1977.

Chapter 5

Planning for Childbirth Education

In the nursing process model, planning seems to be merely one of four equally weighted phases. In actual fact, planning is the essence of professional functioning and is the determinant of whether the desired effects will be achieved in the most expeditious way. It cannot be accomplished without adequate assessment but superlative assessment is useless data unless it is used to plan individualized care.

PLANNING PROCESS

Planning is a logical process that follows a linear progression. Needs determined from assessment data dictate desired outcomes. Outcomes studied within client capabilities dictate approaches to achieving the outcomes. The approaches dictate the criteria for evaluating the achievement of the outcomes and the suitability of the approaches. Viewed as a whole, this process is essential to being able to do more than offer a "cookbook" approach, which is the same no matter what the audience wants or needs, with no room for change because evaluation is either done on a personal preference basis or not all (Fig. 5–1).

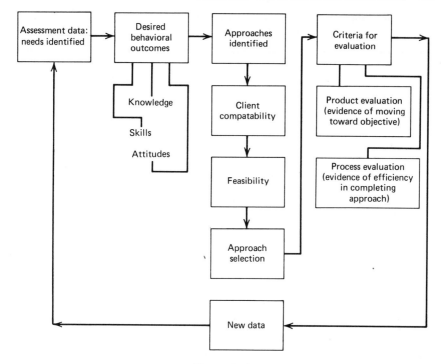

Figure 5–1.

The planning process.

The Planner's Philosophy

At this point, it is important to return to a phrase that accompanied the introduction of the nursing process model: "Professional nurses operate from individual frames of reference that represent personal beliefs, values, commitments and points of view that are culturally developed."[1] The childbirth educators will be influenced by their own frame of reference, which can have an impact on how they will develop an overall childbirth education program. For that reason, it is important to try to identify one's own frame of reference or, in educational terms, philosophy. Many people have only a vague idea of what they believe; others have clearly dogmatic beliefs. But before assessment can be used for planning, it is essential that the planner be able to state clearly those beliefs that make up the frame of reference that will provide

1.   College of Nursing Faculty, *Nursing Process Model* (Tampa: College of Nursing, University of South Florida, 1974).

themes throughout the educational program. This self-disclosure is not an easy process. It is one of the most difficult things to take pen in hand and commit one's beliefs to the stark reality of ink and paper. Some people will never be able to do that at all. Others will work at it and never be quite satisfied that the statement says exactly what they mean. Others will be able to write what they believe and use it consciously in building their program for parents.

An Example of a Personal Philosophy

The following philosophical statement was written in 1968 at the beginning of the author's career in childbirth education. It seems just as relevant today and continues to serve as a guide for working with parents.

> It is my belief that education for responsible parenthood has its foundation in the individual upbringing experienced in the background of the parent. The foundation can be augmented in that period between conception and delivery when the parent is probably most receptive to information about pregnancy and the future of the baby. It is my belief that it is the *right* of every parent to experience the highest possible form of physiological and psychological achievement in the process of childbearing from the time of conception through the postnatal adjustment to new life circumstances. It is my further belief that all unnecessary trauma resulting from fear and ignorance should be avoided through adequate education and counseling. My philosophy is an outgrowth of my belief that health care is a basic human right. I further believe that the dissemination of adequate, comprehensible information is a basic part of health care as well as being essential to the promotion and protection of health. The maternity cycle is a normal process. But the normalcy of the process does not negate the value of education as a preparation for the most healthful continuation and completion of the process. Finally, I believe that every family has the *right* to experience the highest form of achievement in the birth of their child that is possible within their own limitations and goal.

A philosophical statement relevant to childbirth education must be an organized iteration of the individual's beliefs about 1) health, 2) parenthood, and 3) education, because the beliefs held about these three constructs will have an impact on the plan the childbirth educator is able to develop. It is individual beliefs that make one person's program different from those of others.

Planning and Needs

Having defined a philosophy, the childbirth educator can then look at the needs identified in the assessment phase. In planning the overall course, the needs of particular import are those that have been delineated for the community. It means that the assessment information must be reviewed and these questions asked again:

- For whom is the program to be planned?
- What kind of socioeconomic picture does the community present?
- What aspects of their heritage will influence the way the expectant parents view the childbearing process?
- What can they be expected to bring to class with them as strengths and weaknesses?
- What are their perceived needs for childbirth education?

While all these questions are important, probably the place to start the planning process is with the last question: what are their perceived needs for childbirth education? Yura and Walsh indicate that compliance with a plan is more assured when the client has perceived the need as a need.[2] Therefore, starting with the needs the clients themselves have identified and building a program gives the program itself a better chance for success and satisfaction. This approach is one way to organize.

Establishing a Priority of Needs

The process of organizing begins by listing the needs that have been identified. The list is then viewed as the basis for the program. In order for it to provide direction for program development, the items in the list of needs must be put in order of importance. To do this, the educator must identify a theoretical frame of reference so that there is a rationale for priority. Maslow's hierarchy of needs is one frame of reference that serves well as a basis for establishing priorities.[3] Erickson's Eight Stages of Man is also a possible basis

2. Helen Yura and Mary B. Walsh, *The Nursing Process,* 2nd ed. (New York: Appleton-Century Crofts, 1973), p. 78.
3. Abraham Maslow, *Motivation and Personality* (New York: Harper & Row, 1954).

for establishing priorities.[4] There are many more, and one is limited only by one's own knowledge in choosing a frame of reference that can be used for this purpose. Whatever is chosen as the number one need for the community then becomes the main focus of the childbirth education program. The other needs are not ignored. They are incorporated in the program within the thrust of the priority emphasis.

Writing Objectives

Once the needs have been assigned priorities, objectives can be written. Objectives are educational tools. In many institutions they have been misused and abused.

Educational Objectives

Educational objectives are tools that describe the end goals of the educational program. They can be expressed as program goals, or outcomes of the program—at the end of the program, the teacher will have taught . . . Or they can be learner objectives, or outcomes for learner behavior—at the end of the program the learner will . . . Many teachers can write program goals, that is, they can state clearly what they will be teaching. Not nearly so many can write learner objectives, which clearly state what the learner will be able to do upon completion of the program. Both kinds of objectives are important. The former provides the teacher with direction for preparing the material to be taught. The latter are the basis for evaluation of whether the learner has learned.

The Three Domains

The three domains of human behavior form a framework for writing educational objectives.

	COGNITIVE DOMAIN[5]
	Knowledge
THINKS	Comprehension
	Application
	Evaluation
	Synthesis
	AFFECTIVE DOMAIN[6]
	Attending

4. Eric Erickson, *Childhood and Society* (New York: W.W. Norton, 1963), pp. 247–74.
5. Benjamin Bloom, ed., *Taxonomy of Education Objectives: Handbook I: Cognitive Domain* (New York: David McKay Co., Inc. 1956).
6. David R. Krathwohl, Benjamin Bloom, and Bertram B. Masia, *Taxonomy of Educational Objectives: Handbook II: Affective Domain* (New York: David McKay Co. Inc., 1964).

FEELS Responding
    Valuing
    Organization
    Characterization
    PSYCHOMOTOR DOMAIN[7]
    Perceptions—senses
DOES Set—readiness
    Guided response—with help
    Mechanism—can do alone
    Complex overt act—automatic

Some examples of objectives written for these domains might be:

Cognitive domain. At the end of his program the learner will:
 Identify basic anatomy and physiology of labor and delivery;
 Explain the mechanisms of labor;
 Relate the techniques of the psychoprophylactic method to the sensations of labor.

Affective domain. At the end of this program, the learner will:
 Accept parturition as a normal process;
 Practice self-help tools at home regularly until delivery;
 Verbalize a commitment to prepared childbirth as a family experience.

Psychomotor domain. At the end of this program the learner will:
 Perceive the difference between muscular tension and relaxation;
 Consistently use breathing basics;
 Use controlled relaxation on verbal cues;
 Execute breathing techniques combined with controlled relaxation automatically.

To summarize objective writing, it is a process that grows out of discovery. Based on the teacher's discoveries about self and the population to be taught *and* based on what the teacher *knows* about pregnancy, labor, and delivery as well as educational process, the teacher sets objectives. There is a distinction between input from the consumer and abdication to them. Parents sometimes know what they want; sometimes they have only a vague feeling of what they need; sometimes they turn to the educators and say in effect "Teach me everything." The planning of a sound educational program is the responsibility of the teacher. It will reflect the parents' input within the teacher's frame of reference (Fig. 5-2). In this way, the program will best meet the shared needs of expectant parents and the perceived needs of the particular group in the community for whom the program is designed.

7. Elizabeth J. Simpson, "The Classification of Educational Objectives: Psychomotor Domain," *Illinois Teacher of Home Economics,* Winter 1966–67 (reprints available).

Figure 5-2.

Priorities in prenatal education. (From Joyce Roberts, "Priorities in Prenatal Education," *JOGN Nursing*, **5**:17–20, May/June 1976. Reprinted with permission of author and Harper & Row, Publishers.)

PRENATAL TEACHING GUIDE (1st through 32nd weeks)

1st–12th Weeks	12th–24th Weeks	24th–32nd Weeks
Woman more concerned with herself, physical changes with pregnancy, and her feelings about the pregnancy.	Woman has usually resolved the issue of the pregnancy and becomes more aware of the fetus as a person.	Woman becomes more interested in baby's needs as a corollary to her own needs now and after birth.
Changes that are normal for pregnancy	Growth of fetus	Fetal growth and status
Breast fullness	Movement	Presentation and position
Urinary frequency	FHT	Well-being—FHT
Nausea and vomiting		
Fatigue	Personal hygiene	Personal hygiene
EDC—calculate and explain.	Comfortable clothing	Comfortable clothing
Compare with uterine size	Breast care and supportive bra	Body mechanics and posture
Expectation for care	Recreation, travel	Positions of comfort
Initial visit	Vaginal discharge	Physical and emotional changes
Subsequent visits	Employment or school plans	Sexual needs/changes. Intercourse
Clinic appointments	Method of feeding baby	Alleviation of
Need for iron and vitamins	Breast or bottle	Backache
Resources available	Give literature re methods	Braxton Hicks contractions
Education	Avoidance or alleviation of	Dyspnea
Dental evaluation	Backache	Round ligament pain
Medical service	Constipation	Leg ache or edema
Social service	Hemorrhoids	Confirm infant feeding plans
Emergency room	Leg ache, varicosities, edema, cramping	Prepare for breast or bottle feeding
Danger signs	Round ligament pain	Nipple preparation
Drugs, self-medication	Nutritional guidance	Massage and expression of breast
Spotting, bleeding	Weight gain	Preparation for baby
Cramping, pain	Balanced diet	Supplies
	Special nutritional needs	Household assistance
		Danger signs
		Preeclampsia
		Headache, excessive swelling, blurred vision
		Tubal ligation (papers prepared ahead)

Figure 5-2. (continued)
PRENATAL TEACHING GUIDE (32nd week to term)

32nd–36th Weeks	*36th Week to Term*
Woman anticipates approaching labor and caring for baby after birth.	Woman should feel ''ready'' for labor and for the assumption of caretaking responsibilities for baby, even though she may feel anxious about both of these as well.
Fetal growth and status	Review signs of labor (or teach)

Personal hygiene
  Positions of comfort
  Rest and activity
  Vaginal discharge
	Review or continue instruction re relaxation and breathing techniques

Alleviation of discomfort
  Backache
  Round ligament pain
  Constipation or hemorrhoids
  Leg ache or edema
  Dyspnea
	Finalize home preparations
	Anticipation of hospitalization
	  Admission (ER and labor admitting room)
	  Examination, IV, shave, possible enema
	  Care in labor
	  Medication and anesthesia available
	  Postpartum care
	  Supplies needed: bra, personal items, money
	  May have two visitors
	  Tour of maternity unit

Recognition of ''false labor''—Braxton Hicks contractions How to cope and ''practice'' with these	Confirm plans to get to hospital; care of other children. When to go and where
Nature of ''true labor''—signs. Difference between ''bloody show'' and bleeding	Consider family planning needs

What happens during labor
  Labor contractions and progress
  What she will experience
	Emergency arrangements
	  Precipitate delivery
	  Premature rupture of BOW e' or s' contractions
	  Care away from home
	  Vaginal bleeding

Relaxation techniques	

Breathing techniques
  Abdominal
  Accelerated pattern
  Panting and pushing	

Involvement of husband or significant other	

Provision for needs of other children
  Anticipation of baby
  Care for children at home while mother is in hospital	

DEVELOPING APPROACHES

Once objectives have been formulated, approaches for achieving those objectives can be developed. Curriculum development grows directly out of the objectives. Each program will be unique because it reflects the unique combination of the teacher's philosophy and the community's particular needs. And yet, each program will have commonalities with other programs for expectant parents because expectant parents share many common needs during pregnancy.

Objectives and Approaches: What to Teach

One approach to developing a curriculum for a childbirth education program is to sit down with objectives in hand and write a content outline that includes all the material that should be covered to achieve the objectives. Three points to bear in mind are those made by Gorman:

1. Learners are motivated to learn when they can associate new learning with what they already know (known to unknown);
2. Learning is built from the simple to the complex;
3. Learning is enhanced when the learning situation permits application of learning in as realistic a situation as possible.[8]

The content outline, therefore, is a logical progression from simple to complex ideas, moving from subjects known by the learners to new subjects. The easiest way of doing this is to identify the most important concepts and make a list of them. Arrange the list in order of logical progression (known to unknown, simple to complex). Then take a clean sheet of paper for each major topic on the list and use the topic for a title across the head of the page. Underneath the heading list a phrase that describes each of the ideas, concepts, or skills needed to complete the section of the outline described at the head of the page. These phrases should reflect the common needs of expectant parents and the specific needs assessment of the target population. When the sections are complete, it is time to stop progress to double-check. All the sections can be laid out side by side. The educator then takes the objective statements and compares them with the outline sections, asking the question: In which section is this objective partially or completely approached? This

8. Alfred H. Gorman, *Teachers and Learners: The Interactive Process of Education* (Boston: Allyn & Bacon, 1969), pp. 13–14.

comparison gives the planner a chance to be sure that all objectives are included. It is also an opportunity to reevaluate the progression of the outline. What may have seemed clearly logical in the early planning stages may seem out of step when the total outline is developed. By having the sections on separate pieces of paper, the planner is less likely to feel the "etched in concrete syndrome." For some reason it is much easier to switch the order of two pieces of paper than it is to reorder a sequentially numbered continuous outline. For that reason, writing out a formal outline really is the last step in this phase of planning. The outline itself is only a tool, a guide for the teacher. Although major sections should not be left out, it is not a cookbook recipe to be followed step by step ad infinitum. Implementation, to be discussed at length in Chapter 6, will frequently be determined by a particular class of parents. Some will require every minute item of information identified for the outline: others will gloss over whole sections lightly and concentrate on other sections as needed. Critical evaluation must be built into the planning process so that the outline remains relevant. Childbirth education, like other areas of nursing, is dynamic and is reshaped by the changing needs of parents. A relevant outline in 1960 would have to be revised to be relevant today. Who can say what the needs of parents will dictate in the year 2000? The only safeguard is to build in heuristic capability in every outline created. That is the planning process.

Planning Strategies: How to Teach

Once the teacher has decided what to teach, the obvious questions are: How? There are many "hows." How long should the course take? How long should each class be? How should each topic be presented? How is the best way to get the learner actively involved? Some of these questions will be answered by the obvious needs of the population. The course must be completed before the pregnancy is. The expectant mother has real problems sitting for more than one hour at a stretch. These kinds of obvious considerations will influence the planning of such things as when to register for a course—a six- or eight-week course should probably be started no later than the very beginning of the third trimester of pregnancy. Each class session should probably be broken into hourly segments. While it is usual to plan for two-hour classes, a comfort break halfway through is almost imperative.

Decisions about teaching approaches or strategies are not always so obvious. In reviewing the content outline, the educators need to consider the weight of each segment or unit in the overall plan. For some units the material can be presented quickly and is usually grasped readily. For other material, more time must be planned to achieve the unit objectives. These objectives

Figure 5–3.

Writing objectives.

Sample

Main objective	Unit objectives
The learner will recognize the basic anatomy and physiology of labor	The learner will:
	1. recognize pelvic terminology
	2. identify uterine segments
	3. locate pubic symphysis
	4. define uterine contraction
	5. relate uterine location to location of other pelvic organs

are no less important than the overall course objectives and need to be spelled out. They are, in fact, the specific learning outcomes within the unit that will assist the learner in meeting the larger objective (Fig. 5–3).

In addition to the specific outcomes planned for each meeting, there are components of instruction that will also be important in planning for each class. Rheba de Tornyay identified six components of instruction:[9]

1. Using reinforcement
2. Using examples (models)
3. Using illustration
4. Using questioning
5. Creating set
6. Achieving closure

Reinforcement
Use of reinforcement is a tool for the teacher to employ to encourage student participation or to emphasize important points. Reinforcement is the act of calling attention to a person or idea. It can be achieved by repeating the salient points made or simply by agreeing with what has been said.

Example
Use of examples or modeling is a tool for demonstrating the practicality of what is being taught. It is very effective to have speakers from prior classes

9. Rheba DeTornyay, *Strategies for Teaching Nursing* (New York: John Wiley and Sons, 1971), pp. 3–60.

return to talk to current classes. A new mother is probably the leading expert on motherhood to the expectant mother. Careful screening would therefore be in order if this kind of tool is to be used.

Illustration
Use of illustration is a tool that is commonly employed. In effect, illustrations take abstract concepts and make them concrete by comparing them with some common objects or events with which the learner can relate. Of course, the teacher must select illustrations that are commonly known to the audience.

Questioning
Use of questioning is as old as Socrates. It is a tool for actively involving the learner. Posing questions forces the learner to think of possible answers even if none are actually spoken. When questions are answered, it serves as a feedback mechanism for the teacher to gauge the group's understanding of the material being covered.

Creating Set
Creating set is probably the most important component of education for any learning situation, but most especially for childbirth education. Whether the program is early pregnancy education, preparation for labor and delivery or parenting, the affective domain plays an equal if not greater role in the effectiveness of the overall venture. Creating set is the process by which the teacher communicates an atmosphere that allows appropriate attitudes to develop. For childbirth education the two main attitudes that need to be fostered are, first, the normalcy of the maternity cycle and, second, the confidence in the ability of the expectant parents to assume successfully the role of parent when their child is born. Creating set, therefore, is overcoming prejudices and providing a definite frame of reference for the course. This process may sound very simple, but, that is because most of us are not even aware of our "mind sets." All our lives we grow up in an environment that tells us how to perceive and what the unwritten rules are. This to a great degree influences how people behave, rather like the old saw: "My mind is made up; don't confuse me with the facts."

The following exercises are designed to illustrate mind set. The educator should try to solve them without looking at the answers.

Exercise 1: CAN YOU FIND THE BABY IN THIS DRAWING (Fig. 5–4)? First, look at the drawing and try to decide what it is you see.

Mind sets:
1. The baby will be a drawing hidden in the picture.
2. Signs are usually made of black letters on white space.

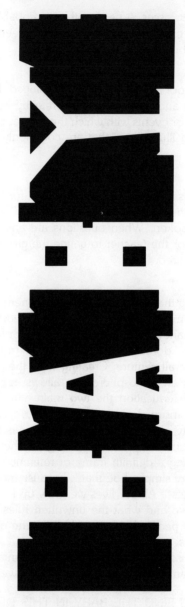

Figure 5–4.
What do you see in this diagram?

Exercise 2: CONNECT THE DOTS (Fig. 5–5)[8]. Without lifting your pencil from the paper, connect the dots with four lines.

Mind set:
• The dots are arranged in a rectangular configuration and the lines are assumed to have to fit within the shape.

Exercise 3: MAKING NINE INTO SIX (Fig. 5–6). With only one line, change the numeral 9 into the numeral 6.

Mind sets:

1. The 6 has to be a Roman numeral.
2. The line has to be straight.

Mind set plays an important part in childbirth education. Parents will have prejudices that need to be discussed; they will bring up old wives' tales that need to be dispelled. The set created for the program can make the program successful by influencing the attitudes of the participants.

Achieving closure
Next to creating set, achieving closure is the most fundamental component of instruction and it is often unplanned. Closure occurs when there is a definable end to the teaching–learning segment. Ideally, teacher and learner reach that point simultaneously. However, sometimes one or the other arrives there first. If it is the teacher, then the learner usually is left with many unanswered questions. If it is the learner, then the teacher may be teaching to an absent audience—even if they remain physically. More often than not, closure is achieved by the clock. Classtime is up and the class ends whether or not teacher or learner have quite finished the business of the day. The master teacher plans for closure and incorporates a closure technique, such as summarizing or forecasting the next segment, as a part of personal teaching style.

Selecting Teaching Strategies
Choosing appropriate teaching strategies is closely tied to the learning objectives and the strengths and weaknesses identified for the population. For example, it would be inappropriate to plan a lecture series for a group of teenage single mothers. Similarly, a totally unstructured, seemingly content-less discussion program for a group of highly educated expectant couples would be equally inappropriate. An understanding of sociocultural influences on education reveals why the teacher would probably lose the audience in each instance. In the former, the "classroom" atmosphere would further

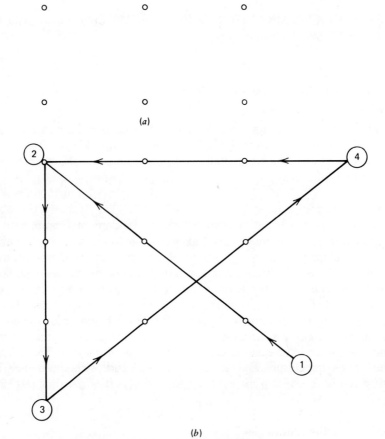

(a)

(b)

Figure 5–5.

Using only four lines, connect these dots without lifting your pencil from the paper. (b) Solution.

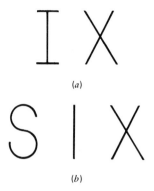

Figure 5-6.
(a) With only one line turn this 9 into a 6. (b) Solution.

alienate these young women who have demonstrated that they are already alienated from the formal educational system. An unstructured discussion program would be a better strategy in meeting their needs not only for information but also for support from an authority figure, the teacher, and from their peers in the group. In the latter situation, highly educated people require precise information and are frequently made anxious by the ambiguity of an unstructured program. For this kind of audience, the strategy of choice would be a combination of lecture and discussion, which provides factual information as a framework from which discussion can arise. The key to the success of a program is the ability of the teacher to assess accurately the particular needs of the intended audience and to remain flexible enough to adapt teaching strategies to those needs (Fig. 5-7).

There are two foci for deciding for or against a particular approach to teaching. Planned approaches need to be considered in light of these two considerations:

1. Is the approach compatible with the learner's assessed status?
2. Is the approach feasible in the circumstances in which the program is being offered?

For instance, teaching breathing techniques may be compatible with the parents' beliefs and learning abilities, but it is not feasible to expect parents to gain any expertise in the techniques if they are demonstrated once in a series of classes whose main focus is general maternity care.

Therefore, when selecting appropriate teaching strategies, the educator should weigh each strategy for compatibility and feasibility as a part of the

Figure 5-7.
PROS AND CONS OF TEACHING METHODOLOGIES.

(Developed by Dr. Albert Smith for the first Regional Conference of the Faculty Development in Nursing Education Project Southern Regional Education Board, Atlanta Georgia, October 16–18, 1977).

Method	Advantages	Disadvantages
Simulation and Games	Facilitate transfer of learning Represent real life processes Engage student in activity Cost less than real life situation Permit failure without real life consequence	Give incomplete view of reality May be too simplistic Lack student accountability May not be effective at higher levels of learning
Mastery Learning	Assigns major responsibility of learning to student Provides teacher with an evaluation on how well students learn Forces student to work harder Reduces duplication in curriculum Provides structure for low-ability students Results in more competent graduates	May be costly, i.e., initial preparation time Results in high attrition rate May be difficult for anxious students Requires new roles for teachers
Experiential Learning	Increases student retention Relates action and concrete events Provides opportunities for relating theory to practice Provides more relevant education	Is time consuming Requires different faculty roles

Method		
Lecture	Is inexpensive Requires less preparation time Covers more content Can be changes easily Is effective	Is uni-directional Encourages intellectual passivity Fails to encourage creativity Has low retention rate
Personalized Systems of Instruction (PSI)	Are viewed positively by students Increase learning Individualize instruction Personalize instruction Reflect higher student achievement	Average higher student Require large amount of time to plan Are not to be used for courses where level of mastery cannot be specified
Discussion	Is responsive to student needs Involves student in learning process Provides wider variety of perspectives Can be effective in changing attitudes Can be effective in learning difficult tasks	Is unreliable in terms of outcomes Is not very effective in conveying content Takes time to develop groups
Audio-tutorial (sic)	Activates several student senses Provides more durable student learning Focuses on student learning not teaching Promotes higher student achievement Is cost effective	Requires large initial investment of time and resources Is not completely self-paced Requires extensive student orientation

selection process. One way to do this is to use a selection chart, (Fig. 5–8) in which the topic to be taught is highlighted. Then, all possible strategies that could be used for teaching that topic are indicated. Each strategy is considered from the point of view of compatibility with the parents' beliefs and learning ability and from the point of view of feasibility given the constraints of the circumstances under which the program is offered such as time, money, and space. In this way there is a rationale for selection. The selection chart can be kept and becomes a documentation of rationale for such time as course revision is contemplated.

Planning for Evaluation

Once teaching strategies have been chosen, the final phase of planning is entered. While not really difficult, it is frequently overlooked or postponed. Planning for evaluation is as important as planning teaching methodology. Evaluation is a continual process although many people treat it as a final test offered as ex post facto evidence that they did what they claimed to do. Evaluation is the process of gathering data for the purpose of making a decision. Criteria for evaluation are the guidelines for data gathering.

Product Evaluation
Educational evaluation looks at two things. First, it looks at the product of education. This kind of evaluation asks the question: Did the learner learn what it was expected that he would? In other words, did the learner achieve the objectives? This kind of evaluation therefore is looking at the effectiveness of the learning situation. Criteria for effectiveness are statements that indicate to the teacher that the learner is moving toward meeting the objective. For example, if the objective states that at the end of the course the learner will identify the basic anatomy of labor and delivery, then a criterion for effectiveness might read: "One week after anatomy and physiology of labor lecture, the learner will correctly name and locate three pelvic landmarks on the birth atlas." This evidence would be an indication that the learner is moving toward the larger objective and probably can be expected to achieve it by the end of the course.

Process Evaluation
The second thing that educational evaluation looks at is the process of teaching–learning. This kind of evaluation asks the question: Is there a better way to teach this material? It looks at use of manpower, material, financial resources, and time. Criteria for efficiency are statements that predict teacher behavior limits in terms of time, money, or material. For example, a criterion

Figure 5–8.

SAMPLE SELECTION CHART FOR TEACHING STRATEGIES.

Topic	Lecture (F)	Lecture (C)	Group (F)	Group (C)	Demonstration return (F)	Demonstration return (C)	Media assisted (F)	Media assisted (C)	Other (Specify) (F)	Other (Specify) (C)	Select
Anatomy of L & D	Y	Y	N no time	Y	N no models	N	Y Birth atlas	Y			Lecture media assisted
Review of birth process	Y	Y	Y	Y			N no funds for films	Y			Lecture group
Contraception	X strong religious objection	N	Y	N	N no models	N	N No funds for films	N			None
Baby care	Y Class time limited	N	N Class time limited	Y	N No models	Y	Y Already own film	Y			Media assisted

F = feasible   C = compatible   Y = yes   N = no

for efficiency might say: It will take the teacher no more than 45 minutes to describe the basic anatomy of labor using the birth atlas. The limit is a best guess based on experience. If it takes longer, the teacher needs to examine why. Perhaps next time, more class time needs to be allotted. If it takes less time, the teacher needs to consider whether all the material has been included that was intended when the estimate was made.

Learner feedback

Learner evaluations are very useful for feedback. Many programs ask for postpartum reports. These are very valuable if taken as part of a whole to determine a pattern. But it must be remembered that each report individually is merely the perceptions of the particular people and offer only one view of a situation, whether ultrafavorable or ultraunfavorable. However, when taken as a part of a whole, it is a tool that can tell a teacher a great deal about points to emphasize more or less in the future.

The other kind of learner evaluation that has been collected is the end-of-the-course reports. The most useful ones are relatively unstructured and ask parents to comment in their own words, especially identifying those areas they would have liked to have done differently or added. Whatever kind of evaluation is to be used, planning for it is an important part of the planning process.

SUMMARY

Planning educational programs is an intellectual process that can make the program of the highest quality if it is carried out logically. Beginning with the identified learner needs and abilities, the planning process applies educational theory to identifying the best way to meet those needs through education. The process follows a logical progression from writing objectives to identifying appropriate teaching strategies to planning for evaluation of both the finished product and the process by which the product has been achieved. Planning is continual and subject to change as new data points to new directions.

BIBLIOGRAPHY

Espich JE, Williams B: *Developing Programmed Instructional Materials*. Belmont, Calif, Fearon Publishers, 1967.

Gagne RM: *Conditions of Learning*, ed 2. New York, Holt, Rinehart & Winston, 1970.

Goetting T: Teaching Resources for Childbirth Educators, *JOGN* **6:**3, May/Jun 1977.

———— Update: Resources for Childbirth Educators. *JOGN* **6:**6 Nov/Dec 1977.

Jones P, Oertal W: Developing Patient Teaching Objectives and Techniques: A Self-Instructional Program *Nurse Educator,* Sep/Oct 1977.

Joyce B, Weil M: *Models of Teaching*. Englewood Cliffs NJ, Prentice-Hall, 1972.

Junior League of Seattle: *A New Life: Prenatal and Postpartum Teaching Guide*. Seattle, Wash, Junior League of Seattle, 1977.

Lowell SL: Patient Education and Self Care: How Do They Differ. *Nursing Outlook* **26:**3, March, 1978.

Meier PP, Mead LP: A Nurse's Guide to "How to Parent" Manual, *JOGN* **7:**1, Jan/Feb 1978.

Murray R, Zentner J: *Nursing Concepts for Health Promotion*. Englewood Cliffs, NJ, Prentice-Hall, 1975.

Nunnally D, Bird IS: The Clinical Specialist—Link Between Theory and Practice, *JOGN* **4:**2, Mar/Apr 1975.

Popham WJ, Baker EL: *Systematic Instruction*. Englewood Cliffs, NJ, Prentice-Hall, 1970.

Raths L et al: *Values and Teaching*. Columbus, C. E. Merrill Company, 1972.

Trow WC: *Teacher and Technology*. New York, Appleton-Century-Crofts, 1963.

Chapter 6

Implementing a Childbirth Education Program

Like assessment, implementation is an active, observable process. Unlike planning and evaluation, which are largely intellectual activities, implementation entails the use of cognitive, affective, and psychomotor skills in direct client activities. To use an old cliche, implementation is the proof of the pudding—the step in which the childbirth educator can test in the real world the plan that has been developed.

RESOURCES FOR IMPLEMENTATION

There are several considerations for successfully implementing an educational plan. Most come under the heading of resources—human, financial, and material resources are all important in the successful achievement of program objectives.

"Who shall teach?" is an essential question. The auspices under which the program will be taught will influence the atmosphere of the program. The sources from which money for the program will be available will definitely affect the nature of the program's implementation. And, finally, how available and appropriate the material resource are can affect whether a program meets its stated objectives.

HUMAN RESOURCES: WHO SHALL TEACH

The question of who shall teach childbirth education is one that is fraught with emotional conflicts. Historically, in this country, the teachers of childbirth education were frequently women who had had a "successful" birth experience, whatever that meant. However, as there are many ways to approach the education of expectant and new parents, and as preparation for parenthood should be an integral component of antepartal care, professionals have slowly moved to take control of this important area of client service. "Why," you may ask, "emphasize professionals?" The answer is threefold. First, the professional practitioner, physician or nurse, has a perspective of the childbirth process that stems from experience with both the normal and the abnormal. The nonprofessional has limited exposure and tends to generalize from personal experience. Secondly, the professional has an understanding of the health care delivery system and the various roles with which the expectant couple will have to intermesh. The nonprofessional does not have a firsthand understanding of this working relationship and can only present the picture as she thinks it may be. Third, the broad background in the supportive sciences that is inherent in medical and nursing education and synthesized in the practice of the professional is often essential in the classroom. The role of counselor is frequently adjunct to the childbirth education course, which if properly planned and executed covers the maternity cycle, including the needs of new parents (Fig. 6–1).

Childbirth Perspective

The childbirth process is transitional in the life of the family. The family approaching the birth of a child has many needs that can be anticipated as a part of the normal maturational crisis of childbearing. However, the birth of the child is not the climax, the culmination, nor the end goal. All too often in the past, parents were led up to the delivery as if it were the ultimate with little or no preparation for dealing with the trials that occur in the adjustment period after the birth of the baby. Preparation for childbirth is the process by which the parents are given tools to cope with the stresses of labor and delivery. But the professional childbirth educator recognizes that the new family will also have needs growing out of its changing family structure and will help the family members anticipate these needs and seek appropriate professional assistance when they are not able to deal with them effectively alone.

Childbirth Educator Preparation

Childbirth education, regardless of the particular approach or emphasis of the course, is an identifiable educational process requiring specific knowledges and skills. Yet, the specific knowledge and skills are not necessarily a part of the basic education of the nurse or physician, although each may have had some exposure to prepared parents as part of the obstetrical experience. More than a passing acquaintance is necessary for the nurse to assume the role of professional childbirth educator. (Very few physicians have sought to participate in the childbirth education program in a role other than guest speaker or advisor.) Legal advisors are very clear about the relationship between background and practice:

> Once the nursing profession has accepted a function as one falling within the sphere of nursing, then each nurse who carries out the

Figure 6–1. (a)

The Role of the Childbirth Educator. (Sasmor, JL: *"Role of the Childbirth Educator,"* N.A.C.O.G. Technical Bulletin on Childbirth Education. Reprinted with permission of publishers.)

The professional childbirth educator has three major functions in the childbirth team. First, in relation to the expectant parents, the childbirth educator serves to provide factual information, to assist in the development of self-help tools for use during labor to instill in parents reasonable expectation for role behavior for all members of the team involved in the process of childbirth and newborn care, and to assist the parents in the transition of the parenting role.

Second, the childbirth educator functions as a coordinator between the desires of the expectant parents and the realities of the labor situation. In this role, the childbirth educator can be a resource person to both parents and staff or change agent if long-term planning is possible.

The third function of the childbirth educator is the relation to the professional members of the childbirth team. With these people, the childbirth educator functions as a collaborator. In this guise, the childbirth educator can use her professional background to assess physiological or psychological problems that can be brought to the attention of the physician or labor nurse so that individualized care can be planned when the parents are admitted to the hospital. Likewise, in this guise, she is open to receive feedback from the physician, labor nurse or postpartum or nursery nurse regarding individual couple performance or definite trends in behavior that point to a need for change in teaching.

Figure 6-1. (b)

The Childbirth Educator's Role

Team Members	Antepartum	Intrapartum	Postpartum
Mother	Resource person. Teaches relaxation breathing, comfort measures. Assesses physiologic and psychological state.	Properly trained parents are able to function with sufficient independence so that they require only intermittent support from available labor staff. Occasionally, the husband-coach may be unable to be present at the labor and the childbirth educator acts as monitrice.* Whether paid or voluntary, the monitrice is not a hospital employee and does not relieve the hospital staff of its responsibility for monitoring the safety of mother and baby. Likewise, the monitrice has no authority to dictate medical or nursing intervention deemed necessary for the safety of mother and/or baby. If monitricing is a regular practice in an institution, specific policies must be developed to govern responsibilities and behavior as well as stipulating the qualification of those eligible to monitrice. This should be a joint medical–nursing committee decision, based on awareness of the needs of the local situation.	Follow-up visit to assess early parenting adjustment.
Father	Establishes role of coach. Helps develop team concept and effort. Assesses ability to work with wife and to cope with stress.		Follow-up report to obtain feedback on delivery experience.
Physician	Communicates any unusual findings relative to mother's status or father's ability to cope.		Solicits feedback on individual couple performance.
Labor nurse	Communicates class performance. Predicts area where support of nurse is needed for mother or father.		Solicits feedback on individual couple performance.
Postpartum nurse	Communicates any unusual concerns that mother or father have expressed that might influence postpartum adjustment.		Solicits information about postpartum adjustment.
Nursery nurse	Communicates any concerns parents may have that might influence early parenting.		Solicit information about newborn status.

*Monitrice is the French word used to designate the trainer who becomes the labor coach in traditional Lamaze settings.

function must obtain the systematic instruction needed for her to acquire the necessary knowledge and skill to support her practice.[1]

This legal advice is just as true for the practice of childbirth education as it is for the administration of medication. Nurses who assume the teaching and counseling roles are as accountable for their professional actions as those who perform the more visible tasks of nursing. Unfortunately, it has been assumed, all too often, that a nurse with knowledge of labor and delivery, or worse yet a nurse from any field who has had a baby, is ready to teach expectant parents. This assumption is erroneous and explains why the quality of expectant parent education is so lacking in uniformity. The nurse who wants to teach expectant and new parents needs to gather the tools of education to add to the nurse's professional skills.

Where can a nurse who wants to teach expectant parents gain the needed preparation? The proper place for nursing education is in schools of nursing. Fragmented, unrelated workshops are useful only as augmentation. Apprenticeship-type learning was long ago recognized as a poor educational model in nursing education and it is haphazard at best. The placement of programs to prepare childbirth educators should be in schools of nursing. The nature of the education is that it builds on the basic nursing education and therefore is rightfully placed with the schools' offerings for continuing education. Until these kinds of programs are generally available, the preparation of childbirth educators will remain in question.

Teaching Teams

With the growing acceptance of family-centered maternity care and increased father participation during pregnancy, labor, delivery, and the postpartum adjustment period, there is also an emerging teaching pattern that combines the nursing expertise of the professional with the warmth of attitude and team spirit of family-centered maternity care. Successful husband–wife team teaching of childbirth education was first reported by nurse psychologist and childbirth educator, Sandra O'Leary, PhD, in 1970 to the Third World Congress of Psychosomatic Obstetrics and Gynecology. In a culture where teachers are often women, the husband–wife team is a model that can help overcome the basic culturally learned reluctance that fathers have to taking an active role in supporting their wives during the maternity cycle. In addition,

---

1.   Irene Murchison and Thomas Nichols, *Legal Foundations of Nursing Practice* (New York: Macmillan Co., 1970), p. 82.

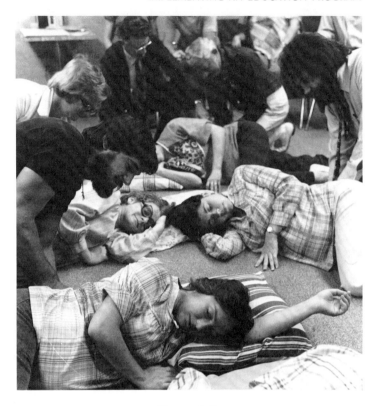

Figure 6–2.

In classroom practice, the male team-teaching member (man in dark jacket) is invaluable to the support of the coach as he learns his role. (Used with permission.)

the husband–wife teaching team working together in the educational process serves as a role model for husband–wife cooperation, which in a sense gives the expectant parents permission to follow their inclination to share the experience of childbearing (Fig. 6–2).

Couple-to-couple childbirth education is a valid teaching strategy, but as is valid for any strategy, if it is to work to its full potential, it must be understood and undertaken as seriously as any other tool the childbirth educators uses. For the team teaching effort to succeed, it is essential that both members have a clear understanding of the goal to be accomplished and their particular contribution to meeting the goal. Therefore, as part of the teaching plan, the specific strengths of each team member must be identified and built in to the approaches. However, for successful execution of the plan, there is one absolute. The team members *must* be compatible. Nothing is more confusing to learners than to have team members correct each other in class. Nor is there anything less likely to build trust than to have team members trying to upstage each other or undermine each other's positions.

Husband–wife teaching teams are composed of equal partners—neither one is more important than the other even though their contributions may be quite different. Each has something vital to offer the participants in the course. One may be the recognized "expert" with many titles and offer the class knowledge. The other may have no applicable titles but offers the class attitude and style which go a long way toward establishing and maintaining interest and self-confidence. It is the smooth meshing of these two contributions that results in the high-quality program that leaves parents feeling knowledgeable and able to cope with the experience of parenthood.

Guest speakers

Occasionally, the childbirth educator will invite a guest speaker: a professional such as an obstetrician or a labor nurse, or former students to share their particular experience. Guest speakers must be carefully chosen so that their presentation does not undermine the childbirth education program because of conflicting ideas or unfortunate personal experiences.

FINANCIAL RESOURCES

The circumstances under which a childbirth education program is offered will communicate many unspoken messages to the parents attending. The circumstances will be determined largely when the childbirth educator makes a basic economic and philosophical decision—to be either a childbirth educator in private practice or an employee with a responsibility for teaching childbirth education. A seemingly straightforward decision, it is one that is often not even weighed by the childbirth educator before the choice is made. The advantages and disadvantages of each program setting bear careful consideration in light of the childbirth educators' own anticipated response to dealing with the results of the decision: economic, legal, philosophical, and interpersonal for both client and professional.

Hospital-based Childbirth Education

Hospital-based childbirth education programs in which the childbirth educator is an employee of the hospital have several intangible advantages. First, holding classes at the hospital helps to eliminate some of the mystique surrounding the hospital as an institution. Being able to relate to the childbirth educators within the institution can increase the parents' confidence before hospitalization; in effect, the repeated visits to the hospital to attend relatively stress-free classes help to desensitize the parents. Second, the hospital setting for the childbirth education program enhances communication between the childbirth educator and the other nursing personnel who will serve the parents during their stay in the hospital. Finally, as an employee of the hospital, the childbirth educator has ready access to the parents for follow-up counseling after the delivery of the baby.

The disadvantages of the childbirth educator being an employee of the hospital are also primarily intangible. The program may be restricted to reflect the philosophy of the institution rather than the philosophy of the childbirth educator. When these restrictions become a matter of patient rights, the childbirth educator is faced with a definite conflict between the role of agent of the hospital and that of parent advocate. Secondly, artificial rules created for the convenience of the hospital such as dress codes and other stereotyping markings may well be at variance with the childbirth educator's attempts to build a warm, accepting milieu. In fact, they may act to erect unnecessary barriers to communication between the parents and the childbirth educator.

On a more personal level, the employee status does offer financial and job security as long as the childbirth educator is willing to stay within the rules and restrictions imposed by the institution.

Community-based Childbirth Educators

Another employee situation that is possible in some communities is through the local childbirth education association. Since the association is community-based, whether the actual course takes place in the hospital depends largely on the group's relationships with the hospital and the hospital's policies on maternity care. If the program is taught in the hospital by the childbirth education association, the setting will have the same advantages and disadvantages as if the program were taught by a hospital employee, except that the childbirth education association usually charges the fee for the course and pays the instructor's salary. If taught in the community, through a community college, an adult education center, or some other community service agency, the program does lose the advantage of frequent hospital contact. However, in some areas this may be preferable to the program emasculation that would be required by moving it into a hospital setting. The group then provides the childbirth educator with support and services needed to coordinate a community-wide childbirth education program.

Private Practice

The alternative to employment for childbirth educators is to enter private practice, offering service directly to the parents in return for a fee. This status also has advantages and disadvantages. As a practitioner outside the established structure, the childbirth educator has to make a special effort to maintain communication with the other professionals in the health community. Physicians need to be aware of what the program is. The hospital personnel need to know what they can expect the parents to know and do.

In favor of private practice, the childbirth educator can offer a program that reflects personal philosophy and accept the role of client advocate without jeopardizing an employee status. To do this, however, the educator must know the legal boundaries of practice in the state as expressed by the nurse practice act in force. Second, the educator must be reconciled to assuming the role of business person in establishing a private practice, because the program must be self-supporting if it is to continue to be offered.

For most nurses, who have usually been employees for their entire career, the very idea of being—or becoming—an entrepreneur is loathsome. This reaction is in part a result of fear, fear of failure in a new and unknown role. Another reason that nurses scorn private practice has to do with tradition from which the profession came. Nursing has long been considered a "calling" and has been invested with all kinds of mystical and romantic features that totally divorce it from reality. Nursing is a professional service commanding a just financial compensation. This fee for service is further hidden in the employee role when the salary is unrelated to the service rendered. Nurses who endorse the romantic "calling" notion find it abhorrent to associate their practice with the business of charging and collecting fees. Nevertheless, fee for service is the basis of the salary they are paid.

Because these attitudes are often unconsciously held and represent habitual, traditional thinking, those who hold these points of view may not even be aware of their existence, yet feel hostile toward nurses who decide to go into private practice.

The surroundings in which an educational program is offered will greatly affect the overall impression that the parents have of the program itself (Fig. 6–3). There is no right setting for every single childbirth educator. Any choice represents a compromise between the advantages and disadvantages to the individual practitioner. Each childbirth educator should consider how her

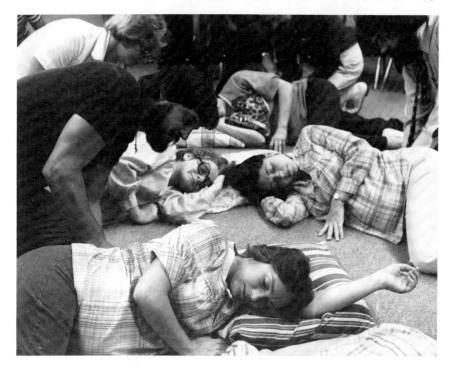

Figure 6–3.

Crowded conditions for practice in a hospital-based class. (Used with permission.)

choice will affect her. There is only one strong recommendation relative to circumstances of teaching. Childbirth education is a professional service. Admittedly, it gained its first momentum as a grass roots movement. However, the time has come to move childbirth education out of the living room of the childbirth educator. The original intent of providing a homey quality has outlived its usefulness if one examines the teaching–learning process (Fig. 6-4). Further, the interruptions of one's family and one's pets are distractions from the educational process.

Many childbirth educators who have grown up with the movement look upon the childbirth education program as a source of small but regular income that requires relatively little time and effort away from home and family responsibilities. These educators feel that the expense of classroom rental would take away too much from their income. While this view may meet the needs of the teacher, it is less than fair to the learners. The home setting reduces the atmosphere of the program to that of any social gathering,

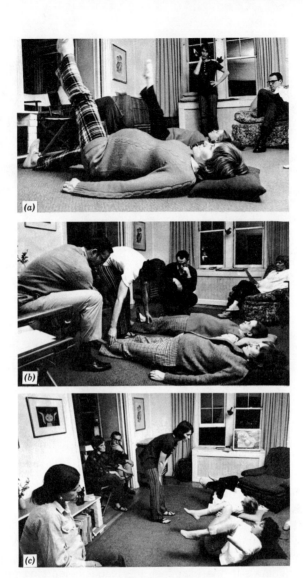

Figure 6–4.

Classes in a home setting. (a) Simple body-building exercises are helpful for strengthening back and abdominal muscles. Wives practice raising and lowering the leg slowly, while inhaling through the nose. Knees are straight; toes are pointed. (b) Neuromuscular control exercises help keep the body relaxed during labor. While husbands give commands to "contract" and "relax" leg and arm muscles, wives learn to turn focus away from abdominal pain. (c) The final lesson teaches a technique for labor-room pushing. With the back at a 45° angle, legs held firmly at the knees and the breath held, wives practice correct use of the muscles which will help with expulsion. (From "Childbirth by the LaMaze Method—Mother-to-Be and Infant Care," *American Baby*, Fall 1970. Reprinted with permission of publisher.)

in which the main purpose is to be entertained rather than to gain knowledge and skills.

Childbirth education is serious business; it is not a social occasion. As such, childbirth education programs deserve a setting that will communicate their main purpose to the learners.

COMPARISON OF PRIVATE PRACTICE AND EMPLOYEE PRACTICE

FACTORS	PRIVATE PRACTICE	EMPLOYEE PRACTICE
Economic	Program must be self-supporting	Program may be subsidized to meet its capital and ongoing overhead
	Personal income tax status complicated—requiring direct payment to IRS for Income Tax and FICA	Withholding and FICA prepaid as part of payroll plan
	Self-employed not eligible for unemployment insurance	May be eligible for unemployment if agency contributes
Legal	State Nurse Practice Act may restrict or prohibit nurses in private practice	As an employee, the childbirth educator can assume teaching role as part of assigned duties
	Many insurance companies do not recognize nurses in private practice for liability insurance	Personal and institutional liability cover teaching activities of employees
Philosophical	Program can accurately reflect the philosophy of the childbirth educator	Program restricted to reflect the philosophy of employing institution
Client relationships	Childbirth educator may have difficulty in establishing credibility initially	Childbirth educator is seen as authority figure by virtue of employment status.
Professional relationships	Childbirth educator may be perceived as an "outsider" or a threat to established practice	Childbirth educator is usually accepted by other professionals as long as institutional limits are observed.

Need for Funding Sources

Education, if it is to be of any value to the participants, costs money to produce. When the cost of education is hidden in the tax dollar and education is universally available to children, then it is often hard to make the public understand that the educational process is an expensive one. Childbirth education is no exception.

Funds are needed to produce a quality childbirth education program just as they are needed for other programs. The childbirth educator preparing and teaching the program is applying professional knowledge and skill and should receive fair and just compensation for time and effort. Funds are needed to make ancillary resources, such as a childbirth education library, available to those who participate. Purchase and maintenance of the hardware and software used in mediated instruction also needs to be considered. The need is real and if not acknowledged and met results in a program that is only adequate at best.

Direct Payment of Fees

Various sources of funding for childbirth education are possible. One obvious source is the client. In private practice, the childbirth educator sets what is considered a reasonable fee for service and the client is expected to pay the fee. A rough rule is that the fee is approximately 10% of the prevailing obstetrical fee. Many childbirth educators do adjust their fee if the client's situation so warrants. Many organizations such as childbirth education associations and hospitals that employ childbirth educators also charge a fee. However, as some of their expenses are absorbed the institutional fees are often well below those charged by the private practitioners.

Indirect Payment of Fees

Some hospitals offering a childbirth education program do not charge the client a direct fee but consider the program as a patient service and budget for this service. This is usually a part of the nursing budget if there is no discernible patient education budget. In these situations there is no fee but, of course, as a part of the budget is passed along to the client in the long run.

Many communities offer the public the opportunity to participate in childbirth education programs at little or no direct cost through the local community college or adult education center. Offered through community services, adult education, or continuing education, these programs are supported by the tax dollar.

Third-party Payment

There is a possible source for funding of childbirth education in th
Third-party payment has in the past been reserved for physician services. It is
only very recently that nursing services have begun to be recognized by
third-party payers. If a National Health Insurance Program for Mothers and
Children becomes a law, then there is a definite possibility that a case could
be made for third-party payment for childbirth education as a form of anticipatory guidance, reduction of risk, and preventive mental health. Thus
childbirth educators need to be aware of pending legislation and should
consider supporting the legislation that is in the best interests of their clients.

MATERIAL RESOURCES

The use of library resources, films, slides, and other media in the implementation of a childbirth education program can be a big asset. However, media, no
matter how well produced, should never be used to replace in-class teaching.
Media should be used to present graphically, to emphasize visually, or to
reinforce what is being taught. They are not a replacement for poor teaching.

Selecting Media

The key to selection of media is the plan for the program. It is imperative that
the media be selected to meet the objectives and *not* that the objectives be
changed to suit the media available. To do a good job of this, the childbirth
educator will need to preview media to locate the ones that best fit into the
program. One approach is to read the latest edition of the *Film and Record
Directory* (from the International Childbirth Education Association, 1414 NW
85 St., Seattle Washington 98117), and order all media appropriate to the
objectives of the program for preview. This step enables the childbirth
educator to decide if in fact the film, filmstrip or record does exactly fit her
program.

Another approach is to contact distributors directly to request information
that they have available about the media that they distribute, and then order
for preview directly from them.

Still another approach is to contact a national clearinghouse such as the
Health Education Media Association (PO Drawer 54189, Atlanta, Georgia

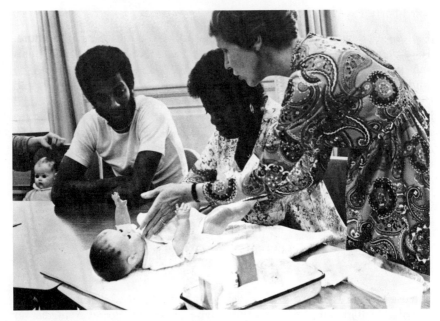

Figure 6–5.

Hands-on activities call for hands-on media. Childbirth educator teaching parenting skills. (Photo courtesy Maternity Center Association, New York, N.Y.)

30308).HEMA can direct the educator to sources and possibly in the long run become a regular resource to the educator for locating media, not only for classroom use but also for her own continuing education.

Developing Media

Sometimes even an exhaustive search does not produce exactly the media to fit the objectives of a given course. It may fall to the childbirth educator to create the media desired. It is not uncommon for the childbirth educator to make charts that collate material from different classes in a series so that the charts in fact act as a summary of the information.

Similarly, while it is not legal to reproduce slides copyrighted by someone else, it is often necessary to combine sets of slides that have been purchased to achieve the course objectives.

Several childbirth educators have created material for their own teaching which they have reproduced and made available to others. Margaret Gamper (627 Beaver Rd. Glenview, Illinois 60025 of the Midwest Parentcraft Center) has done just that with her Labor and Delivery Charts. Another such example is the *Father's Labor Coaching Log and Review Book* (Jett Publications, PO Box 16159, Tampa, Florida 33687). This pocket-sized book was developed because there was no handy source for prepared fathers to take with them into the hospital setting to review quickly or to make their notes on labor progress.

To the childbirth educators who see a need and are willing to act to fulfill it, there are no limits to this kind of creativity, except those that might exist in the minds of the educators themselves.

For those who wish to create slides, tapes, or combinations, the National Medical Audiovisual Center (Atlanta, Georgia), which is supported by the Department of Health, Education, and Welfare may be a resource, provided the request comes from groups that meet their specifications. At the very least, they can provide a directory of media currently available.

SUMMARY

Implementing the plan in putting into action the goals and objectives of a program depends on careful consideration of human, financial, and material resources. The childbirth educator must carefully weigh the advantages and disadvantages of the private practice versus employment status in terms of the educator's own personality and ability to cope with the outcomes of each. Examination of funding sources is necessary to build a full program that can supply adequate material resources such as childbirth education library, films, slides, charts, and other teaching tools.

BIBLIOGRAPHY

――――― Definitions of Nursing Titles *JOGN* **7**:1 Jan/Feb 1978.

American Nurses Association: *Three Challenges to the Nursing Profession.* Kansas City, Mo, ANA, 1972.

American Nurses Association: Congress on Nursing Practices, *Nurse–Practitioner, Nurse–Clinician and Clinical Nurse Specialist.* Kansas City, Mo, ANA, 1974.

American Nurses Association: Commission of Economic and General Welfare, *Third Party Payment for Services of Independent Nurse Practitioners.* Kansas City, Mo, ANA, Jan 24, 1974.

Ashley J: *Hospitals, Paternalism and the Role of the Nurse.* New York, Teachers College Press, 1976.

Auerbach A: *Parents Learn through Discussion.* New York, John Wiley & Sons, 1968.

Baker BA: The Assertive Nurse Practitioner, *The Nurse Practitioner,* **3**:2, Mar/Apr 1978.

Brown K: The Nurse Practitioner in Group Practice, *Nursing Outlook* **22**:108, 1974.

Clark A: *Leadership Techniques in Expectant Parent Education.* New York, Springer, 1973.

Clauson JP: Nursing Leadership of Expectant Parent Discussion Groups, *JOGN* **2**:3, May/Jun 1973.

Cogon R: Practice Time in Prepared Childbirth, *JOGN* **7**:1, Jan/Feb 1978.

Davis F: *The Nursing Profession.* New York, John Wiley & Sons, 1966.

Kinlein ML: Independent Nurse Practitioner, *Nursing Outlook* **20**:1, Jan 1972.

Lewis EP: The Programmed Mother and the Nurse Practitioner, *Nursing Outlook* **26**:3, Mar 1978.

Lysaught JP: Nursing Education as it Affects Specialty Nursing Care, *JOGN* **3**:1, Jan/Feb 1974.

McAbee R: Rural Parenting Classes, *American Journal of Maternal Child Nursing,* Sep/Oct 1977.

Mauksch I, Young PR: Nurse-Physician Interaction in a Family Medical Care Center, *Nursing Outlook* **22**:2, Feb 1974.

Murray BL: A Case for Independent Group Nursing Practice, *Nursing Outlook* **20**:1, Jan 1972.

Nuttleman D: Development of the Role of Nurse Health Educator in a Private OB/GYN Medical Practice, *JOGN* **5**:5, Sep/Oct 1976.

Rill RD: Nurse Health Educator, *JOGN* **6**:6, Nov/Dec 1977.

Roberts S: *Behavioral Concepts and Nursing through the Life Span.* Englewood Cliffs, NJ, Prentice-Hall, 1978.

Sloan L: What Business Structure Is Best For You? *American Journal of Nursing,* Oct 1975.

Subrin L: The Business Aspects of Private Nursing Practice, *JONA,* Sep 1977.

Sundeen SJ et al: *Nurse–Client Interaction: Implementing Nursing Practice.* St. Louis, C. V. Mosby Co, 1976.

Zahourek R et al: *Creative Health Services: A Model for Group Nursing Practice.* St. Louis, C. V. Mosby Co, 1976.

Chapter 7

Evaluating Childbirth Education

Evaluation is the hallmark of any excellent educational program. It is the source of information that allows the program to change and grow in response to the changing needs of the clients. It is the source of new data that make changes relevant. Part of the planning process is to develop criteria for evaluation that serve as standards against which the actual outcomes, both teacher and learner behavior, can be gauged (Fig. 7–1).

CONCEPTS OF EVALUATION

If evaluation is seen as a process around which change develops, then it loses some of its awesomeness as a final proof of merit. Traditionally, in the American educational system, evaluation has been used as a rite of passage that determines personal destiny in many lives: final examinations, college entrance board examinations, and even state board examinations for entry into professional practice. It is no wonder that once most people leave a formal educational setting, they stay as far away from "tests" as they can in their day-to-day lives. In planning for childbirth education, it is thus wise to keep in mind the adult perception of testing. It is not logical to eliminate the evaluation process, however, because it is a necessary source of information upon which the professional can and should base decisions.

121

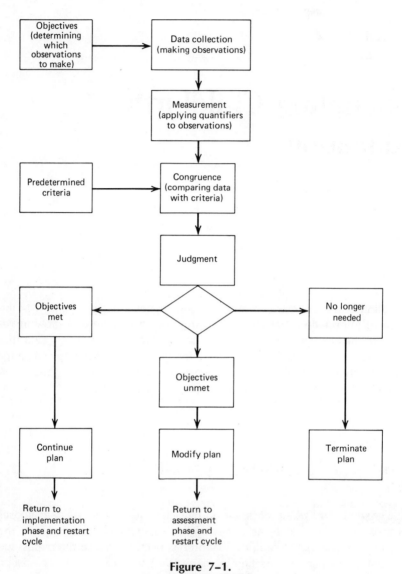

Figure 7–1.

The evaluation process.

There are three concepts of evaluation especially pertinent to the childbirth educator. They are measurement, congruence, and judgment.

Measurement

Measurement is the process of gathering data using quantified descriptors. For instance, if time is being measured, the descriptors are numbers of minutes, hours, days, etc. If cost is being measured, the descripters are dollars and cents. Therefore, educational objectives are criteria for evaluation that must be expressed in quantified terms as well as being stated in observable behavior.

Congruence

Congruence is the process of comparing the gathered data with the predicted outcomes to determine to what degree the desired outcomes have been achieved. For instance, if an objective states that "the learner will correctly identify foods from the four food groups recommended in the diet for a pregnant woman" and the actual outcome is that the learner can identify only three correctly, the finding would be that the learner partially met the objective, having achieved 75% of the stated outcome. Since most educational standards accept achievement at the 70% level or better as satisfactory, this level may be a realistic one for the childbirth educator to set. However, what is considered an acceptable level of performance is at the discretion of the person who is setting it. The childbirth educator may think that certain knowledges or skills are so important that the learner should be expected to perform at the 100% level. For example, in the interest of infant safety, an objective might state that "the learner will correctly demonstrate the proper handhold for lifting a newborn each time lifting is attempted." Acceptable level of performance then would be demonstration of the proper technique every time the skill is tried.

Judgment

Judgment is the process of using the data gathered and analyzed as the basis for making a decision. There are actually only three possible decisions that can be made based on the evaluation data: to continue with the plan as it is; to modify the plan; or, to terminate the plan (Fig. 7–1). The basis for making these decisions is quite logical and depends entirely on the data gathered and analyzed as part of the process of evaluation. If the data reveal a high level of congruence between outcome behavior and objectives, then it can be assumed that the plan is sound, that it is meeting the needs of the learner population. In this instance, the appropriate decision is to continue with the plan and, therefore, the childbirth educator would return to the implementation phase and, using the same plan again, implement and evaluate until data indicate that the objectives are not being met. When the data indicate that the objectives are not being met, that leads to the second possible decision, which is to modify the plan. In order to make any changes in the plan, it will be necessary to reassess the needs of the clients to see if it is possible that the clients themselves have changed. Situational changes that alter the needs of the clients to the extent that the program objectives must be changed can occur in very short periods of time. If the reassessment reveals that the objectives are still relevant to the needs of the clients, then the approaches used should be reassessed to see which strategies are effective and which need to be discontinued or altered. If the reassessment reveals that the objectives are no longer relevant because the needs of the clients have changed, then the only appropriate decision is to terminate the plan, partially or completely. It is most likely that over a period of time, the childbirth educator will terminate portions of a plan while continuing other portions so that a total program evolves. In this way, the childbirth education program remains dynamic, responding to the needs of the clients.

MODES OF EVALUATION

The two modes of evaluation identified in the chapter on planning are *product evaluation,* which relates to the effectiveness of the program in meeting the stated objectives, and *process evaluation,* which relates to the efficiency of the selected approaches. In other words, product evaluation focuses on the learners' abilities and process evaluation focuses on the teacher's abilities. The learners' abilities should be measured in terms of the stated objectives; the teacher's abilities should be measured in terms of the stated approaches to meeting the objectives. Sources of the data for evaluating product include both the teacher and the learner as well as the members of the childbirth team who relate to the learners during the maternity cycle. Sources of data for evaluating process also include both the teacher and the learner as well as any others involved in the actual presentation of the program (Fig. 7–2).

Figure 7-2.

Evaluation modes.

PRODUCT	PROCESS

Focus:
  Learner behavior
	Focus:
	  Teacher behavior

Reference:
  Objectives
	Reference:
	  Approaches

Sources of data: • Teacher/observer • Learner • Childbirth team	Sources of data: • Teacher/observer • Learner • Media recordings
Tools: • Pre-post paper and pencil testing • Anecdotal records • Checklists • Narrative reports • Rating scales • Teacher-led discussions • Team-member conferences • Written team feedback	Tools: • Checklists • Discussion flow charts • Discussion participation scales • Sociograms • Tape recordings (process recoding analysis) • Unstructured/structured end-of-course evaluation form

Teacher-Learner Evaluation

Teacher-learner evaluation is the most traditional approach to evaluation. In this relationship, the teacher makes observations about the learner's behavior to determine whether it indicates that the learner is meeting the stated objectives. The obvious disadvantage of this kind of evaluation is that its accuracy depends on observational powers and the arbitrary judgment of the teacher in making the evaluation.

Also certain areas of learning remain hidden if the evaluation is done in a haphazard manner. This is a particular phenomenon of adult education, in which the learner tends to learn best that which has personal relevance. The evaluation of learner, therefore, should probably be approached using a variety of tools, in order to minimize the subjective distortion that can occur when a teacher uses only one tool that relies only on personal observation.

Teacher Evaluation Tools

Pre/post Paper and Pencil Testing

As stated previously, written examinations are usually very threatening to the adult learner. This tool is nevertheless a useful means of gathering information if test-taking is approached in a way that reduces the personal threat. The answer, simply enough, is to assure anonymity. The information gathered about the client group as a whole is as important for program evaluation as the personal data gathered for individual evaluation. Since the purpose of evaluating is to gather data in order to make decisions about the program, it would seem that program evaluation would be more pertinent, that is, data about the learning that occurs in a group of clients rather than the individual learning that occurs. With this end in mind, a pre- and posttest can be developed and administered. If the clients are invited to participate, anonymously, on the basis that the tests are being administered to see if "the teachers are really teaching what they think they are," most adults will participate willingly. The tests themselves become a learning device if the learners can score their own tests as correct answers are revealed. A bonus in teaching is the results of the pretest. Administered at the beginning of a course, it can pinpoint those areas of content that are strongest or weakest for the group, which helps the teacher plan what content to emphasize. The results also serve as the baseline data against which the results of the posttest can be compared. It is expected that the scores of the group as a whole would improve by the end of the course. Items for the tests should represent critical areas, representative of the course objectives. The analysis of the test results should include a discussion of the overall change as well as the change item by item. These results then give the teacher a reasonably fair appraisal of cognitive learning and an opportunity to identify areas of least effectiveness in the content presentation. When learners score the posttest themselves, the test itself serves as a review of material covered in the course and gives the students an opportunity to see how they have done and how much they remember, without the pass/fail connotation.

Anecdotal Records

Anecdotal records serve mainly as a memory aid for the teacher. During the course of a childbirth education program, many parents express concerns or exhibit behavior that may indicate predictable problems. For example, the expectant mother who invariably directs class discussion to her previous labor experience, which she admits was frightening and unpleasant, is probably excessively anxious about the upcoming experience and will need additional reassurance and support. The parents who reveal that they have lost a baby also need special attention. These kinds of things are often disclosed in a class discussion and, if the childbirth educator has an active practice, it is difficult and sometimes impossible to remember such details, let alone associate them with the correct parents and respond with the individualized attention that will help to meet their needs.

Figure 7–3.

A sample of an anecdotal record for a preparation for labor class.

Anecdotal Example 1

Client's Names: Martha and Steve Parsons	EDC: 7/12
Program: Preparation for Labor	Doctor: Cohen

Class session	Comments
1	Made no comments—difficulty relaxing
2	Husband–wife team work well together with relaxing; spoke of last delivery—sedated
3	Relaxation OK; slow breathing OK; shallow breathing too deep
4	Shallow breathing improved—OK; expressed concern about baby and cord—last baby had to be resuscitated
5	Delivered early 6/30—parents and baby OK
6	

Anecdotal records help the childbirth educator to recall the clients' needs and to provide client-centered educational experiences. They serve solely as means of data gathering; anecdotal records do not in themselves evaluate anything. The examples in Figures 7–3 and 7–4 indicate the kind of data that anecdotals can be used to collect.

The comments on the record in Figure 7–3 do not evaluate the learners except to point out special areas on which the childbirth educator can then focus at the next session, thus providing special help or reassurance as needed.

The comments on the record Figure 7–4 are not unusual for a family in which there is dysfunctional parenting. The baby in this case is at least in danger of being understimulated and sensorally deprived and at worst a possible candidate for child abuse if he continues to live with his parents. This kind of record would merely serve as a memory aid when the childbirth educator contacted the pediatrician or public health department for a referral on behalf of the baby.

Exactly what the childbirth educator chooses to include on the anecdotal record will depend on that part of her observations she considers important. The notes should be short—just enough to convey the main idea. For the most part, the notes should be observations, not inferences.

Figure 7–4.

A sample of an anecdotal record for a parenting class.

Anecdotal Example 2

Clients Names: Maureen and Dave Richardson		EDC 5/30 (Delivery Date)
Program: Parenting		Doctor: Young
Class session	Comments	
1	M. very agitated; D. no comments; baby in carrier whole class; when fussy, pacifier put in mouth	
2	M. refers to baby Michael as "it"; rarely seen to look at him, even when handling	
3	M. came alone tonight; D. to football game; M.'s mother babysitting; M. chatted more than usual; seemed gayer	
4	absent	
5	absent	
6	M. came with baby; no supplies; baby wet and crying; ignored; changed with our diapers—handles impersonally	
7	M. came alone; during class M. stated that she did not want the baby—that she had got "caught"; baby with grandmother	
8	absent	

Checklists

The simplest way to record the attainment of a skill is to use a checklist. This tool is only an indicator of the presence or absence of the skill and offers no information about the quality of attainment. However, lists are easily constructed and simple to complete (Fig. 7–5).

For the list shown in Figure 7–5 skills were identified in order of presentation by week. The double X indicates that the topic has not yet been covered, and, therefore, that the parent could not be expected to have attained it. To use a checklist such as this one, the childbirth educator need only put a plus or minus sign in the appropriate box by week. One checklist is kept for each client.

Rating Scales

An alternative to checklists that provides a more qualitative evaluation record is the rating scale. The rating scale has the advantage of being able to show progress as well as skill attainment. The example of a checklist in Figure could easily be converted to a rating scale by substituting a weighted value for the plus or minus in recording. One way to do this is to allocate points for levels of achievement, such as:

- 0–Cannot do skill at all
- 1–Can do skill with help
- 2–Can do skill correctly without assistance

Figure 7–5.

A checklist sample.

Preparation for Labor Skills

Week	1	2	3	4	5	6
Posture						
Comfort positions						
Physical fitness						
Controlled relaxation						
Slow chest breathing	XX					
Shallow breathing	XX					
Transitions breathing	XX	XX				
Pushing in labor room	XX	XX				
Pushing in delivery room	XX	XX				

Each person is then evaluated each week and an ongoing record of achievement is maintained. It is ideal if the person is earning all 2s by the final weeks of the course.

Another kind of rating scale provides progress reports and comparative information. In this kind of scale both desired behavior and undesired behavior are identified. The scale then provides information that allows the childbirth educator to identify both strengths and weaknesses and thereby individualize the experience to the needs of the client.

For this type of scale, it is probably more useful to use a five-point scale to stand for:

- 0–Never (not at all)
- 1–Rarely (less than 10% of time)
- 2–Sometimes (11–25% of time)
- 3–Usually (26–75% of time)
- 4–Always (more than 75% of time)

The exact allocation of percentages in the definition of the points is set by the person who develops the scale. The settings are arbitrary and have no absolute meaning except as defined for use with the rating system. However, if the scale is used by more than one rater, all raters must agree on the definitions and use the scale with a high level of consistency or the reliability of the tool will be in question.

When a rating scale such as the one shown in Figure 7–6 is used, it would be ideal if the client showed an identifiable trend toward higher ratings on the positive skills and lower ratings on the negative skills.

Teacher-led discussions

Because of the strong emphasis on the group discussion method of teaching for the various forms of childbirth education courses, the teacher-led discussion is a common tool for evaluating cognitive and affective achievement. In order for this to be effective, however, the teacher must have used planning time to reidentify the specific objectives and predetermined criteria that will be indicators of achievement. Broad opening statements and leading questions serve as the strategy for eliciting responses from the clients. The outcome of such discussions does not usually give definitive data on individual achievement but it does alert the teacher to areas of confusion and unanswered questions. This kind of information is invaluable, especially when the course is structured so that each class builds on the information presented in preceding classes.

Learner Evaluation Tools

Narrative Reports

Unstructured narrative reports allow the learners to express their particular response to the use of the skills learned in the course. These have been used most often as "postpartum" reports, describing the clients' actual experience and providing feedback on points of procedure that may have changed or

Figure 7–6.

A rating scale sample.

Parenting Skills Rating Scale

Week	1	2	3	4	5	6	7	8
Skills: *Positive*								
Cuddles baby								
Strokes baby								
Talks to baby								
Looks at baby								
Responds to cry								
Negative								
Does not hold								
Ignores cry								
Refers to baby as "it"								
Is repulsed by body functions								
Does not see anything to like about the baby								

that ought to be added to assure the parents the maximum anticipatory guidance possible in the circumstances.

The use of narrative reports as an evaluation tool should be considered carefully. First, the tool is only as good as the person reporting. With that understanding, the teacher really ought to consider the source, that is, consider the report in the light of other tools that have been used such as anecdotal records or rating scales. Also, each class has a personality all its own. The respondents will reflect the class personality in their reports as well as their own experience; the teacher should consider the reports in the context of the class performance. An example of an actual class report is shown in Figure 7–7.

Finally, narrative reports should be considered from a broad perspective as a source of feedback. A popularity contest is not being held—not all parents

Figure 7–7.
A sample postpartum report form.

POST PARTUM REPORT FORM   Please return to: J. Sasmor. PO Box 16159
Tampa, Fl. 33687

Parent Information:

Names: *Wes & Lori F.*

Address: Telephone:

Which pregnancy?   1   ②   3   4   more. Any unusual problems during pregnancy?
bladder infections

Would you say your overall experience was satisfying? *yes*   Which techniques worked

best for you?   Were you together the entire time?

Baby Information:

Name: *Christopher F.*   Sex: *male*   Birthday: *May 29, 1976*

Height: *22 inches*   Weight: *9 lbs 14oz.*

Did the baby have any unusual problems?   Explain. *Not after delivery. A
C-section was decided upon when it was discovered that Chris' head
would not turn down for delivery.*

BIRTH REPORT:
In your own words describe your experience as completely as possible.   Use
extra paper if necessary.

Mother's Report: *Even though an unplanned C-section was used for
delivery, the breathing techniques were invaluable. I had a very
rapid labor in the early stages but the breathing and pushing in
the delivery room was of great assistance. The practice during the
last night of class was a great help. I had no medication until I
had been in the delivery room pushing for an hour and, then, the
panting came in "very handy" until they were able to give me medication.*

Father's Report: *The classes were very helpful in bringing my wife
and me to the point of "experiencing" our second birth together.
Although I was not permitted in the delivery room, I felt much
more a part of the whole process by being my wife's "coach" at
home during the last two months of pregnancy and in the labor room.*

Any additional comments:

will like all teachers or all methods of teaching, especially those that m.
learner think. Therefore, the teacher should not take individual
personally—no credit for all-glowing reports nor blame for reports that ⸹
If the teacher reviews the reports along with other evaluation tools, this iɔ ɪess
likely to occur.

Postpartum Reunions

For many people who lose the narrative report forms or refuse to take the
time to fill them out, another source of feedback is a postpartum reunion. At
this social event, usually sponsored by one of the couples in the class, the
class members can meet and show off their babies. The informal atmosphere
and obvious pride of the parents usually lead to frank disclosures that the
more formal written report sometimes does not reveal. The childbirth educator,
as a silent observer at a reunion, listening to the parents report to each other,
can frequently learn a great deal about their experiences.

Other Evaluation Sources

The other members of the childbirth team—the obstetrician, the labor nurse,
the postpartum nurse, the pediatrician, the nursery nurse—are valuable
sources of information that can be used to evaluate parent performance.
A good way to get this feedback is to request a team member conference for
the purpose of evaluating the performance of the parents, in order to make
the job of the other team members easier. Very few people can resist the
opportunity to have a say in making their own jobs easier. There should be an
agenda for this kind of conference that identifies the kinds of things that the
childbirth educator wants to know and affords an opportunity for the other
team members to give or elicit information that will make them better able to
care for patients and their families. One fringe benefit of this kind of a meeting
is that it allows the team members, including the childbirth educator, the
chance to communicate with each other in a constructive manner.

At least one institution has tried a written team feedback system that seems
to work well. An anecdotal card is created during the prenatal courses that
indicates the courses taken and level of achievement. The card becomes a
part of the labor record and the labor nurse completes the reverse side, which
consists of a brief checklist but provides space for comments. Despite anticipated reluctance, childbirth educators using this system have found that the
labor nurses not only fill out the checklist portion but also take time to add
valuable comments which can serve to improve the program they offer.

PROCESS EVALUATION

The evaluation discussed thus far, product evaluation, has dealt with the learners' achievement of objectives. The other mode of evaluation, process evaluation, which focuses on the teacher's ability to carry out approaches efficiently, is equally important and usually receives much less attention in evaluation plans. As with product evaluation, the process can be evaluated using checklists and rating scales. The components identified, however, rather than being learner skills, are the specific activities that the teacher has planned to carry out for the class being observed.

Group Discussion Evaluation

There are a number of ways to examine the process of group discussion. Each focuses on how things are being done rather than on exactly what is being said. One such system of looking at behavior in a group was developed by Robert Bales (Fig. 7–8). If utilized by an observer over a class session, it would be one way to categorize the kinds of behavior that the teacher as a group leader exhibits—as a primary style and as backup styles.

Another way to look at group discussion as effective teaching strategy is to construct sociograms. Sociograms are diagrams of interaction. In an effective group, as in Figure 7–9, it would be expected that all members would have a chance to voice something and the teacher would be a resource person. For many experienced teachers it is often eye-opening to see a sociogram of a group they have led and become aware of the extent to which they dominate the discussion (Fig. 7–10).

Media-recorded Evaluations

Audio and video recordings of teacher performance can be revealing. Video, in particular, helps teachers identify distracting, unconscious mannerisms. However, the very act of recording may inhibit the spontaneity of the group unless it is done unobtrusively. The value of the recordings depends on how they are used, a fact that is frequently forgotten in the activity of recording and reviewing the record.

Audio recordings are probably the easier to use, partly because once it is announced that the class is being recorded, the recorder is relatively unseen and soon forgotten. Also, the teacher can review the recording privately, as often as desired, because the recording is usually on tape cassette and most

Balos' System of Observational Categories

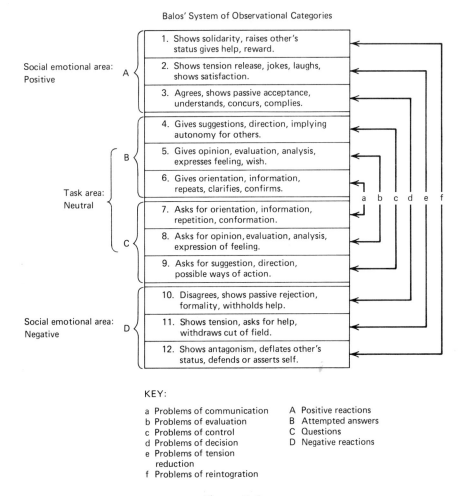

KEY:

a Problems of communication
b Problems of evaluation
c Problems of control
d Problems of decision
e Problems of tension
   reduction
f Problems of reintogration

A Positive reactions
B Attempted answers
C Questions
D Negative reactions

Figure 7–8.

The Bales' Scales. (From Robert Bales, *Interaction Process Analysis,* Cambridge, Mass.: Addison Wesley, 1950. Reprinted with permission of author and University of Chicago Press.)

people have access to a cassette player. Once the teacher gets over the shock of how she sounds on the recording, she can concentrate on the process. The childbirth educator can use a Bales scale or some other tool to evaluate her own performance. For some people, it is easier to understand the process if the recording is transcribed in a process-recording format (Fig. 7–11).

The teacher is then forced to identify the therapeutic or nontherapeutic

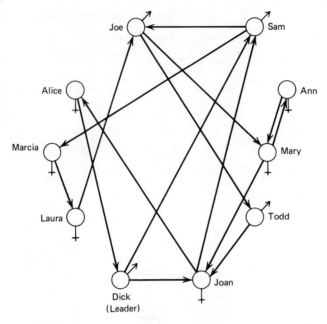

Figure 7–9.

Sociogram of an effective group.

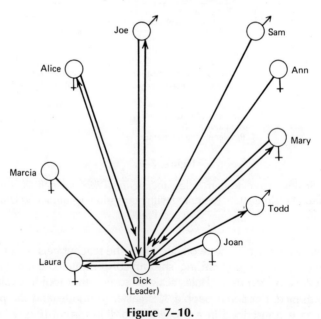

Figure 7–10.

Sociogram of a leader-dominated group.

Figure 7–11.

Form for a process recording.

| Teacher | | Student | | Analysis: |
Verbal	Nonverbal	Verbal	Nonverbal	Open or blocked
T_1		S_1		
T_2		S_2		

techniques that either furthered or blocked communication. Consistent use of blocking techniques will eventually discourage group process and is something that the teacher will want to be aware of and work to eliminate from her style.

Video recordings are less available to most childbirth educators because of the costly equipment. However, if at all possible, at least one video tape of teacher performance would give the childbirth educator a better understanding of the style she uses in the classroom. It helps to eliminate nonverbal distractors—poor posture, suggestive gestures, facial expressions inappropriate to topic, etc. This form of self-evaluation can be very painful to someone who believes herself to be an expert teacher. But it is necessary to improve the quality of teaching.

End-of-Course Evaluation

Regardless of whether a structured or unstructured end-of-course evaluation form is used, most instruments of this type tend to result in a happiness quotient—the information returned has to do with what the clients liked or disliked about the course. As with narrative product reports, these kinds of tools should be reviewed in the context of the group as a whole. It is very easy to become discouraged every time a negative report is received. Sometimes it is deserved and this will show up in the group with many negative reports.

More often, the isolated report is merely the expression of a malcontent whose needs were not met by the course. Somewhere on the form there should be a place where the clients can make suggestions for improving the course. This is a valid way for the instructor to remain in touch with changing needs. However, not all suggestions should be acted upon. All should be considered in the light of the course objectives and those consistent with the present objectives considered for action. Those that are not consistent with current objectives might well eventually lead to the development of a whole new program, or they may have been ideas that had been dropped in the past at the request of other clients. The main point is that the clients should contribute to the evaluation process—both the evaluation of their performance and the evaluation of teacher performance.

SUMMARY

Evaluation is an important part of the educational process. It serves as the basis for decision-making about the future direction of any program. In evaluating childbirth education programs, the teacher should consider both product evaluation and process evaluation, which are equally important. The former refers to the behavior of the client during and after the course as it relates to the stated objectives. The latter refers to the performance of the teacher as it relates to the ability to carry out approaches to meeting objectives. Data collected for both kinds of evaluation provide the direction for continuing, modifying, or terminating the teaching plan.

BIBLIOGRAPHY

Barnard K: Predictive Nursing: The Baby and Parents, *Health Care Dimensions,* 1976.

Bishop B: A Guide to Assessing Parenting Capabilities, *American Journal of Nursing* **76**:11, Nov 1976.

Downs F, Fernbach V: Experimental Evaluation of a Prenatal Leaflet Series, *Nursing Research* **22**:4, 1973.

Geissler EM: Matching Course Objective and Course Context, *Nursing Outlook* **22:**9, Sept 1974.

Gronlund N: *Measurement and Evaluation in Teaching.* New York, Macmillan Co, 1965.

Johnson SR, Johnson RB: *Developing Individualized Instructional Material.* Palo Alto, Calif, Westinghouse Learning Press, 1970.

Mager RF: *Developing Attitude Toward Learning.* Palo Alto, Calif, Fearon Publishing Co, 1968.

Nunnally DM, Aguiar MB: Patients' Evaluation of their Prenatal and Delivery Care, *Nursing Research,* Nov/Dec 1974.

Tyler L: *Tests and Measurements.* Englewood Cliffs, NJ, Prentice-Hall, 1963.

PART THREE

SUPPORT SYSTEMS

Because this entire book is intended as a resource book for nurses interested in childbirth education, it seemed superfluous to include a chapter extolling the virtues of the childbirth educator as a part of the support system of the expectant parents. This section, rather, presents information by and about members of the childbirth team, other than the nurse, in the instances of normal uncomplicated parturition and the special role of the nurse in dealing with two selected exceptions that frequently touch on the childbirth education program.

In Chapter 8 Valin frankly presents the role of the physician in prepared childbirth and offers several cogent suggestions for eliciting physician support.

In presenting the role of the father, Chapter 9, Sasmor strongly maintains a positive point of view regarding father participation, eschewing the common tendency in the literature to describe by exception. This is a masculine point of view drawn from personal experience as a father and seven years as part of a childbirth education teaching-team.

Smith and Lamparelli, in Chapter 10, deal sensitively with the special needs of expectant mothers who are single. Their considerable experience is apparent in the identification of individual and family problems faced by these mothers and in their commonsense suggestion for planning educational programs that take into account both present conflicts and planning for the future.

The final chapter in this section, Chapter 11, deals with a postpartum problem that frequently touches on a childbirth education program—the needs of parents whose child is less than perfect. Taylor developed this chapter with the postpartum/nursery nurse in mind, carefully describing the parent–child bonding sequence and then relating the sequence to the enforced separation with a premature or sick newborn. Special emphasis is given to the need to develop criteria for evaluating the nursing care that will enhance parenting.

Chapter **8**

The Physician and the Prepared Couple

THOMAS J. VALIN, MD

The role of the physician in caring for the prepared couple is a vital one. Without physician support, parents will in all probability be less than successful in achieving their own goals. Parents who have had the experience of participating in the birth of their child can often hardly contain their enthusiasm. It is these exuberant people who will continue to sell these educational programs. However, the fact that a couple has had successful completion of an accepted course and a subsequently rewarding childbirth experience, does not qualify them to make decisions on teaching policies or medical management.

One of the most pressing issues in the growing field of childbirth education is how to obtain maximum physician participation. Without any participation the problem is impossible. With limited participation the program is difficult and frustrating. Physicians are needed; they must be involved—and this is not a simple task.

Author's note. Dr. Valin developed the preceding exposition of the physician's role as a part of a presentation to the First National Summer Working Conference of the American Society of Childbirth Educators in New Orleans, in July, 1972. It is interesting to note that another physician has independently developed a similar treatise in 1978. For a second opinion, read: Joseph T. Anzalone, "The Physician's Viewpoint" in Celeste Phillips, and Joseph T. Anzalone, *Fathering: Participation in Labor and Delivery* (St. Louis: C. V. Mosby, 1978), pp. 18–36.

SECURING PHYSICIAN PARTICIPATION

Physicians who have participated in the childbearing experience of prepared couples do not need to be sold on its virtues. Parents who are well-informed and included in the decision-making about maternity are usually cooperative because they understand the doctor's reasoning. When parents are treated as intelligent adults by their physician, their respect for their doctor and his or her decisions is enhanced by the doctor's attitude. Fear of the unknown and suspicions about unnecessary intervention are minimized when parents can see why a course of action must be taken. This is not, however, an attitude shared by all physicians who care for expectant and new parents. How, then, can the professionals not only stimulate the interest of physicians but encourage their full participation?

There are basically two approaches to soliciting physician participation—the direct and the indirect.

The Direct Approach

One might consider the direct approach or face-to-face confrontation, whereby childbirth educators speak to obstetricians, singly or in groups, trying to persuade them to accept prepared childbirth methods. This is probably the most difficult and the least productive avenue of approach. The reason is that most doctors have been trained in delivery methods other than those involving prepared parents. Very few of the large teaching centers offer the opportunity for residents and interns to deliver infants of prepared parents. In teaching centers most patients are moderately sedated because it facilitates teaching methods when groups of medical students are involved.

Some physicians regard any approach by advocates of the trained childbirth method as a challenge to the tried and true methods they have used for years. They resist third-party intervention. Many physicians are fearful that this new approach to labor and management delivery will require more of their time for the delivery process.

One realizes, therefore, the extreme delicacy of the direct approach. It requires much tact and decorum. It must be attempted by those already on a friendly basis with the physician. A forceful approach is doomed to failure. There is one offshoot of the direct approach that is worthy of consideration. It is the compromise or "Try it, you might like it" approach. It can be suggested that the physician accept a prepared couple, be open-minded, and evaluate the labor and delivery process with a "show me" attitude. Often a physician will be convinced with one prepared delivery.

Another facet of the direct approach involves some truthful subterfuge. A copy of the teacher's manual should be sent to all the obstetricians in a particular area or region. In the manual, information about when to expect to see the doctor during labor and delivery should be explicit and realistic. The student should be advised that the labor room nurse is a competent, well-trained professional, able to manage labor adequately to the second stage, and the doctor will be available when called by the nurse. The point must be made that it is not necessary for the doctor to spend more time with a prepared couple than with any other patient. These points should be under-lined and strongly stressed in class. In this way the doctor knows in no uncertain terms that his or her time is valued. These directives alone will win many a doctor over to at least trying the prepared approach.

Indirect Approaches

There are several indirect approaches to obtaining acceptance of prepared childbirth by physicians. The first approach is through the hospital. In a very subtle manner the administration and the nursing director must be encouraged to give serious thought to allowing prepared childbirth deliveries in their hospital. The first step in achieving this end is to encourage patients who live in the locality serviced by the hospital to write to the hospital requesting that maternity departments be opened to the prepared childbirth programs. Another approach is to interest one of the local women's organizations in the program. In many hospitals these organizations are influential because of their volunteer activities. When the hospital agrees to accept the program it often follows that patients will insist on going there and out of necessity the doctor may consent to try the method. Another entry to the hospital is through a physician already on the staff who is interested in prepared childbirth and may be able to influence the hospital to cater to this group and in so doing encourage other physicians to try the method. In order to satisfy all the needs of the hospital, the childbirth educator should be prepared to furnish copies of the accepted form that releases the hospital from any liability it may have to assume because of the presence of the father in the delivery room. Routine release forms are available for this purpose, and copies should be in every instructor's manual.

The second indirect approach is through the patients. This is perhaps the strongest course of action and many times the most difficult with which to cope. Patients who have had good experiences talk about them and sell the program to others. Word of mouth is the strongest ally. There must be some way to acquaint people with the program before they become patients. They must be knowledgeable enough to seek out a physician who will be willing to provide them with the opportunity to utilize their learned techniques. Instructors are often placed in a delicate position when the student, now seven months pregnant, suddenly finds out that her physician is not in favor of the prepared childbirth technique. The student asks the instructor for advice. In this case honesty is the best policy. If the student has been advised by her physician that he or she really cannot provide her with the type of delivery she wishes and that there are other physicians in the locality who do practice the method, she should be given a list of those doctors from which to choose. As the prepared childbirth program gains strength, the childbirth educator and students will be just as ethically bound as doctor and patient. It might be advisable for local instructor groups, if well organized, to send out a short questionnaire every two or three years asking the obstetricians if they will accept the trained student for delivery. In this way the doctor is given a choice that, if accepted, will place the doctor's name on the list of physicians who take prepared couples for care.

Finally, the third indirect approach is the news media. This is another means of reaching the general populace and one that should be utilized as often as possible. Meetings and film showings should be placed in the newspaper at every opportunity. However, caution is recommended in giving verbal interviews unless the interviewer will allow review of the copy before it goes to print. Otherwise statements could be unintentionally misquoted and result in misleading content appearing in an article.

PHYSICIAN–COUPLE RELATIONSHIP

First, there is no relationship unless the doctor accepts the value of preparation to the couple. Once the relationship is established, there are still real problems unless the doctor understands the ideas and concepts of preparation. Therefore, physician education is important. If it is possible to combine knowledge with sincere interest, we have the ultimate—a physician with experience and the time to offer help when requested. The psychoprophylactic triad needed for success in the hospital is:

1. A well-trained, enthusiastic couple
2. A family-centered hospital
3. An interested, knowledgeable physician

An uninterested physician is able to function and have many successful delivery experiences. But it should not take a sincere, dedicated physician very long to change his or her ideas about this method. Involvement with the couples through their deliveries will win the physician over very quickly. When this happens, the doctor becomes involved and seeks ways in which to provide, better preparation, not just *adequate* care, but the *ultimate* in care. When the new couple is asked, early in their prenatal course, which type of delivery they would like, the physician may slant the discussion toward the prepared approach. This will especially be so if they are vague about the methods available and are not in favor of the woman's being heavily sedated for delivery.

The physician's acceptance of the prepared childbirth concept may also be dependent upon his or her type of practice. Obstetricians practicing in groups, especially in groups of three or more, and those who limit their practice to one hospital may be steered quite easily to the prepared approach because in this type of practice the doctor often spends a greater amount of time in the hospital. Being in the hospital they are more available to the hospital suite and their labor practice. The obstetrician who practices alone often fears that participation in prepared childbirth will require more time and will, therefore, resist all attempts to stimulate his or her interest. Here again physician education is of utmost importance.

With increased experience the obstetrician begins to realize the father's part in prepared childbirth. The doctor becomes aware of his presence and will quickly ascertain his capabilities to perform adequately as a coach in the labor and delivery room. It will be the doctor's responsibility to offer guidance if a father does fail in his supporting role. To do this without harming the close partnership and team relationship takes much tact, but it is not a difficult or insurmountable task. Once again, experience is the best teacher. The physician must not overwhelm the couple in the delivery room. The need for the father's participation in the delivery room, with respect to the experience itself, is very often more valuable to the couple than the delivery itself. It enhances the birth process many times over and makes it a lasting, memorable experience.

SUMMARY

Knowledgeable participation and support by the physician in prepared childbirth is essential if the parents are to have the optimal experience. The prepared couple allows the physician to practice safe and humanistic medicine because they can understand the physician's rationale for necessary decisions in the plan of care. Many physicians still do not accept the need for parent preparation but can probably be swayed in favor of it through direct and indirect approaches.

BIBLIOGRAPHY

Manheimer A: Case Study: Media Coverage of New Treatment Plans, *Perinatology Neonatology* **1**:2, Sep/Oct 1977.

Segal B: A Lamaze Doctor Discusses Father's Role in the Delivery Room, *American Baby,* Aug 1972.

Stern T: Establishing Prenatal Classes in a Small Community, JOGN **2**:5, Sep/Oct 1973.

Chapter 9

The Role of the Father

JAMES C. SASMOR, BS

In a world in which nursing and medicine are usually practiced in an authoritarian and bureaucratic setting comparable at times to a military or governmental milieu, it requires a sharp break with traditional thinking to include the expectant father as a physical and functioning presence in the support system of the expectant mother. Desire and pressure for taking such a step in the United States has been generated and carried out, for the most part, by individuals and groups outside the mainstream of routine obstetrical practice.

For any movement involving practitioners and the public to succeed its time must be right, and this held true for childbirth education. Changes are taking place in the way individuals and couples see their relationships to a changing world. A social environment is evolving in which consumerism and its questioning attitudes are presenting a challenge to traditional methods practiced in many fields. A pressure for satisfactory alternatives that enhance the individual and strengthen the couple is making itself felt.

NEW EMPHASIS ON THE EXPECTANT FATHER

The cause of the father is being championed.[1] Why anyone should present him as an important and potentially useful person in the pregnancy, delivery,

1. Jeannette L. Sasmor, *What Every Husband Should Know About Having a Baby* (Chicago: Nelson-Hall Co, 1972).

149

and nurturing sequence is the critical question. The answer lies in the unique relationship between the partners in those couples suitable for training in father-coached childbirth and cooperative parenting. Now that the opinion that "childbirth is not a spectator sport" has been established, everyone present at labor and delivery should be there because he or she has a definite function for which each has been trained. This can and should be true of the expectant father.

Elements of the Change

Let us consider what is involved in this unusual phrase *expectant father*. What is acting upon and within him that is changing him from a passive figure remote from the action to a participating one? The essence of the difference between the traditionally accepted definitions of the words *mothering* and *fathering* is clear evidence of the mental attitude that guides the actions of many of those involved with parents and as parents.[2] Mothering is regarded as an ongoing activity, fathering as a one-time action. The extent to which fathering can develop into an intermittent activity and then ideally into a continuous activity as an equal partner in parenting, affects human relationships as strongly as the social revolution keyed by modern feminine contraceptives and the changing economic profile of women in our society. Before there can be a widespread change in the actions of individuals within a social structure there must be an attitude reorientation on the part of society. The penalties for excessive variation from traditional ways are high, the opportunities few, if the variations must depend upon the cooperative activities of organized others.[3] With regard to the emerging role of fathering, this means the expectant father must have the opportunity to acquire the knowledge and psychological orientation to make him effective as a constantly functioning member of the *equilateral* triangle of mother, child, father, rather than a triangle in which the father is the narrow side (Figs. 9–1, 9–2).

THE PARTICIPATING FATHER

The decision to be a participating expectant father rather than a passive or alienated one is often not easy. The previously mentioned societal pressures

2. Jeannette D. Hines, "Father—The Forgotten Man," *Nursing Forum*, 1971, p. 189.
3. James Heise, "Toward Better Preparation for Involved Fatherhood," *JOGN*, Oct/Nov 1975, pp. 32–35.

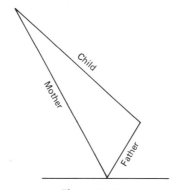

Figure 9–1.

Traditional relationship.

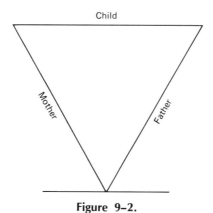

Figure 9–2.

Emerging relationship.

against it must be dealt with, as well as the feelings of inadequacy, the lack of knowledge of what he will be called upon to do, and the guilt of having placed his partner in the endangering, uncomfortable, and distressing situation of pregnancy. The decision, of course, is a joint one. The assurance by his partner that she desires his sharing and assistance in this long and complex journey to a birth is the most important factor in making a commitment that many expectant fathers begin with strongly ambivalent feelings.[4,5] Perhaps

4. Virginia D. Reiber, "Is Nurturing Role Natural to Fathers?" *The American Journal of Maternal Child Nursing,* Nov/Dec 1976, pp. 366–71.
5. Jacqueline Hott, "The Crisis of Expectant Fatherhood," *American Journal of Nursing,* Sep 1976, pp. 1436–40.

the most radical new concept of the family is the inclusion of the expectant father as an active and contributing agent in the actual labor of the mother and the birth of their child.

Society Molds Attitude

The female from childhood on is made aware of and oriented toward the possibility of becoming a mother. By contrast, the male is not oriented toward the possibility of becoming a part of the birthing process. As a matter of fact, he is usually expected to disassociate himself from participation. An example is the response made years ago to a young Navy man who requested leave to be with his wife because she was going into labor: "Your presence is required at the laying of the keel, but not at the launching." This age-old attitude means that creating a prepared father to be part of the birthing team is a two-step operation: first, the negative conditioning must be overcome, and then the positive conditioning and instruction are required.

Attitudes Are Altered by Education

The expectant father as encountered in the first couples class is usually in considerable need of assurance that the role he is assuming is not in violation of the position society, his peers, and his family have set for him or, if to some extent it is, that the benefits that accrue by becoming a new-style, involved father will eventually enhance, not diminish, his masculine standing.[6]

This reorientation in self-image is made easier by presenting his positive activities in terms of his becoming a *coach*,[7] because coaching of athletics is regarded as a highly acceptable masculine endeavor.

Men with a passport into the ultrafeminine area of pregnancy, labor, and delivery have been so far only the obstetricians who, in reality, have become the rulers of the domain. Placing this passport in the hands of the "layman" for his presence in the territory hitherto forbidden by social and medical tradition is accomplished by giving the expectant father preparation in valid and specific tasks to perform in aiding the process of labor and delivery.

The preparation is usually structured as a course meeting once each week for six weeks conducted by childbirth educators. An innovation designed to

6. Barbara Kiernan and Mary Ann Scoloveno, "Fathering," *Nursing Clinic of North America* (Philadelphia: W. B. Saunders, 1977).
7. Jeannette L. Sasmor, *The Father's Labor Coaching Log and Review Book* (Tampa: Jett Publications, 1972).

strengthen the teaching of the expectant father is the male–female instructor team, which offers the advantage of male-to-male communication.

The couple presents an acquiescence form signed by their obstetrician. The content of the psychoprophylaxis course, briefly, is an explanation in simple terms of physiology of pregnancy and delivery, strengthening, relaxing and conditioning exercises for the pregnant woman, and breathing patterns to diminish awareness of sensations of contractions. All the way, the father is taught functions that assist his laboring partner—timing of contractions, observation for unwanted muscular tension, aid in maintaining appropriate breathing patterns, and advised comfort measures.[8] In addition, as a trained observer of his mate, the expectant father also acts as reporter and communicator to the labor nurse and obstetrician. In this regard the effectiveness of the prepared father will depend upon the understanding and cooperation of the hospital staff as to what the prepared couple is trying to accomplish.

The husband's confidence is built as the couple advances through the course and his secureness in the new role increases. When he then has the opportunity to be of definite assistance to his wife and to share as a coach her experience of childbirth, he gains through this positive contribution a stronger emotional bond with mother and child.

The Importance of Both Technique and Confidence

The successful teaching of the psychoprophylactic method of prepared childbirth can be looked upon as the achievement of two separate and distinctly different elements. On one hand there is the conditioning and developing of the physical aspects: the exercises, the breathing methods, the timing practices, as well as the learning of the physiology, birth process, and vocabulary. On the other hand there is the establishment and cultivation in the minds of the couple the belief that this procedure *does work* and that it can, when properly applied, give them the results of a controlled labor and delivery for which they hope and are trained to achieve. It must be emphasized that a negative attitude shown by any staff member may destroy for the couple this essential conviction, that what they are doing can produce the result they desire.[9] The husband-coach is highly vulnerable, because a vital part of his task is to maintain the laboring couple's dedication to the value of the techniques when the stress increases. If properly prepared, he has confidence in the importance of his presence as a contributing member of the

8. *Ibid.*
9. Patricia Huprich, "Assisting the Couple Through a Lamaze Labor and Delivery," *The American Journal of Maternal–Child Nursing,* Jul/Aug 1977, p. 245.

group around his laboring wife. The nurse should recognize the benefits in supporting a competent coach.

Challenges to the Role

Addressing this point, an editorial from a leading journal of nursing states:

> Since many of us in the helping professions are decrying the breakdown of the family structure, it seems somewhat ironic that we often are the very ones who put obstacles in the way of families who want to remain together, particularly in times of stress. While there are many examples of such obstacles in the field of maternal child health, routinely prohibiting fathers from the delivery room seems to epitomize them all.
>
> Why? Because in this day when it is recognized that encouragement from loved ones can minimize stress and maximize one's ability to cope, it seems irrational to prevent a couple from working together during a birth. Yet this is still done on many occasions.
>
> . . . is this a situation in which providers are defending a system that meets their own needs and maintains their authority rather than serving the consumer?[10]

Those practitioners who are resistant to the changes created by having the father present are prone to state that the expectant father is likely to make his presence an undesirable burden on the busy labor and delivery room staff by fainting, roaming, regurgitating, or interfering in a number of other spectacular, distracting, and possibly legally threatening ways. The facts do not confirm this contention.[11,12] Properly prepared expectant fathers take care of their own physiological needs during the hours of labor. They have been instructed to take the opportunities to eat and drink and to relieve themselves and not to exhaust their systems to the point at which physical or emotional stress would make them less than useful. They have also been advised of the possibility of acute emergency situations that are grounds for the physician's directive that they leave immediately and they are prepared to comply. It would be well to

10.   Barbara Bishop, Editorial, *The American Journal of Maternal–Child Nursing*, Jan/Feb 1978, p. 7.

11.   Kathryn Antle, "Psychological Involvement by Expectant Fathers," *JOGN*, July/Aug 1975, p. 42.

12.   Linda R. Cronenwett and Lucy L. Newmark, "Father Responses to Childbirth," *Nursing Research*, May/June 1974, p. 210.

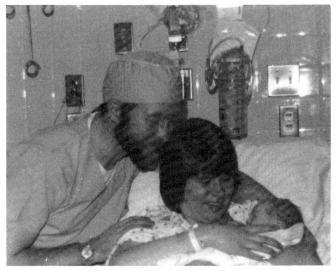

Figure 9-3.

In the Recovery Room immediately after delivery. Note the enfolding behavior—
Sally enfolds Sarah in her arms and Jeff enfolds them both with his arm.

state here that because all team work includes the extremely important
element of interacting personalities it is highly desirable that the physician and
the expectant father make a point sometime early in the pregnancy and
several times thereafter of meeting for purposes of evaluating each other. This
is usually not convenient for either the physician or the father, but it can pay
great dividends in mutual confidence and is invaluable should the going really
become difficult. Similarly the nurse should make some effort to evaluate the
father and to assess how helpful he may be expected to be to the staff and in
what areas they may contribute to what he has to do.

Advantages of Stronger Bonding and Expanded Care

The benefits of having the prepared father present through labor and delivery
continue beyond the birth.[13,14] Research into the psychological area called
"bonding" or "binding" places great importance upon the initiation and

13.   Marcia Gollober, "A Comment on the Need for Father–Infant Post-Partal Interaction,"
JOGN, Sep/Oct 1976, p. 18.
14.   Marshall Klaus and J. Kennell, *Maternal–Infant Bonding* (St. Louis: C. V. Mosby, 1976).

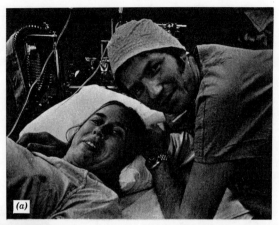

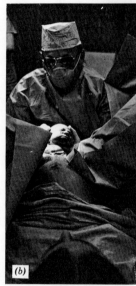
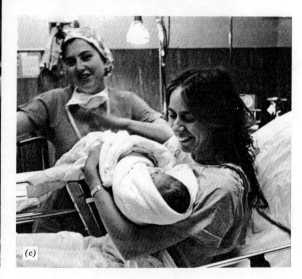

Figure 9–4.

Diary of a Lamaze Father. (a) "Judy and I prepared together for the birth of our child. Here we share a moment together in the delivery room just before the birth." (b) Dad's first view of Sarah. (c) Judy, awake and aware and happy, holds Sarah in the delivery room. (Photographs by Ron Goodman from "Diary of a Lamaze Father," *American Baby*, June 1974. Reprinted with permission of photographer and publisher.)

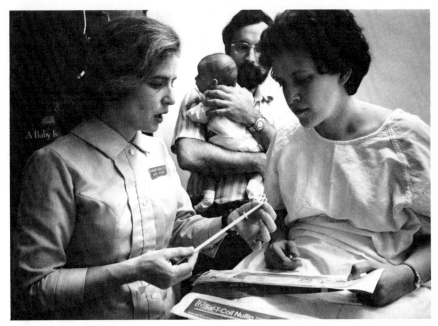

Figure 9–5.

The new father stays interested after delivery. Here this father cares for the baby while the new mother is learning about the options for family planning in an outpatient setting. (Photograph by Robert Goldstein from Margaret Bean, "Birth is a Family Affair," *American Journal of Nursing,* Oct. 1975; reprinted with permission of photographer and American Journal of Nursing.)

strengthening of ties between the newborn and those in contact with the infant. It has been reported that in the first hour of life the neonate has a receptivity to developing these ties that is higher in intensity than in its later development.[14,15] The value of the opportunity for the father to be a touching, holding, communicating presence at this critical time becomes even greater when this is considered.[16]

Having broken with tradition by close and supportive association with his wife's pregnancy, labor, and delivery, the new father now stands on the threshold of a further departure from the usual paternal path. To do this, he has been prepared as a performer of the cleaning, feeding, and comforting

15.   Reva Rubin, "Binding-In In the Post Partum Period," *American Journal of Maternal–Child Nursing,* May/June 1977, p. 67.
16.   M. Greenberg and N. Morris, "Engrossment: The Newborn's Impact upon the Father," *American Journal of Orthopsychiatry,* 1974, pp. 520–31.

activities for the couple's newborn.[17] Just as classes for husband-coached labor and delivery were attended by the expectant father, so were classes in care of the infant. His warm and tender interest in wife and newborn, so satisfyingly given active and useful expression in the pregnancy and delivery-coaching role, now finds its continuity in the application of his recently acquired knowledge in baby care. Again he has mastered a course involving both the development of techniques and the development of confidence. He has achieved a further important step in extending his side of the triangle beyond its heretofore narrow limit.

SUMMARY

A drive for increasing participation and control on the part of a substantial percent of those who comprise today's society is altering the nursing relationship with the expectant father. It is essential that the nurse understand the goals and training of the prepared father. The attitude and conduct of the nurse is a potent influence on the performance of the expectant father as a labor coach and later as a nurturing parent. The benefits to be gained by supporting the expanding role of the father should guide the nurse in this area of practice.

BIBLIOGRAPHY

———— For the Expectant Father. New York, Maternity Center Assn. Pamphlet.

Arnstein H: The Crisis of Becoming a Father, *Sexual Behavior,* April 1972.

Beigner J: Fathering Research and Practical Implications, *Family Coordinator,* XIX, Oct, 1970.

Benson L: *Fatherhood—A Sociological Perspective.* New York, Random House, 1968.

Biller HB: *Father, Child and Sex Role.* Lexington, Mass, Heath Lexington Books, 1971.

Birdwhitsell R: Is There An Ideal Father?, *Child Study* XXXI, Summer 1970.

17.   Ross D. Parke and D. B. Swain, "Fathering: It's a Major Role," *Psychology Today,* Nov 1977, p. 112.

Brenton M: *The American Male: A Penetrating Look at the Masculine Crisis.* New York, Coward McCann, 1966.

Dodson F: *How to Father.* Los Angeles, Najh Publishing, 1974.

Duxbury ML: Maternal Bonding: The Importance of Early Attachment Between Parents and Child, *American Baby,* Sep 1977.

Farrell W: *The Liberated Man.* New York, Random House, 1975.

Goelsch, C: Fathers in the Delivery Room: Helpful and Supportive, *Hospital Topics,* Jan 1966.

Goodman R: Diary of a Lamaze Father, *American Baby,* June 1974.

Green M: *Fathering.* New York, McGraw-Hill, 1976.

Lamb ME: *The Role of the Father in Child Development.* New York, John Wiley & Sons, 1976.

Leonard J: Fathering Instinct, *MS,* May 1974.

Lynn DB: *The Father: His Role in Child Development.* Monterey, Calif, Brooks Cole Publishing Company, 1974.

May KA: Active Involvement of Expectant Fathers in Pregnancy: Some Further Considerations, *JOGN,* March/April 1978.

Meerloo J: The Psychological Role of the Father, *Child & Family,* Spring 1968.

Morton J: Fathers in the DR—An Opposition Standpoint, *Hospital Topics,* Jan 1966.

Norton GR: *Parenting.* Englewood Cliffs, NJ, Prentice-Hall, 1977.

Osofsky J (ed): *Handbook of Infancy.* New York, John Wiley & Sons, 1978.

Salk L: How Great to Be a Father, *Family Health,* Feb 1971.

Schwartz A: *To Be a Father.* New York, Crown Publishing Co, 1967.

Steinberg D: Redefining Fatherhood—Notes After Six Months in LK Howe, *Future of the Family.* New York, Simon and Schuster, 1972.

Chapter **10**

The Single Parent

PAMELA LAMPERELLI, MSW

JANE M. SMITH, RN, CCE

The obstetrical staff is an important part of the professional team that offers services to single mothers. Counselors welcome and depend on reports from the nurse that might help them to be more therapeutic with their clients. Often the patient who has developed a comfortable rapport with her nurse will in fact relate very important facts that the counselors should know. A nurse who deals with single mothers might find it most advantageous if she acquainted herself with the pregnancy counseling agencies and/or maternity homes in the area in which she works. The counselors would be happy to meet the nurses who care for their clients. Any qualified pregnancy counseling agency would be most willing to offer the nursing staff inservice education classes. Sadly, for many single mothers, proper counseling is not always available. If the nurse observes that her patient is not handling the pressures of her pregnancy well, the patient should be referred to a qualified pregnancy counseling agency.

THE SINGLE MOTHER

Today we are meeting not only single mothers but also a large number of women who have been married but for one reason or another are facing this pregnancy alone. These single-parent mothers, many of whom are multiparas, are also considering surrendering their babies for adoption. They

160

have in many cases already given birth to previous children and have been able to enjoy bonding with and nurturing their previous infants. Seeing this particular pregnancy through alone may indeed be extremely difficult for such a mother. A positive, understanding attitude on the part of the nursing staff will be most helpful to her at this time.

Special Problems

Because of the many social pressures and personal rejections that the single mother may be dealing with, she may find it difficult to accept her pregnancy. Any pregnant woman may begin to deal with the acceptance of her pregnancy when she first feels the baby move. If the nursing staff gives her an opportunity to express her feelings about the baby's movements, her acceptance of the pregnancy will be enhanced. Recognizing this newfound fetal activity with the mother and sharing the varied emotions involved would also be supportive.

The single parent who is rejected by her baby's father often has many more anxieties during her pregnancy. Her prenatal visits are very important to her and she looks forward to positive reinforcement about her prenatal progress. For many single expectant mothers, seeing the pregnancy through and producing a healthy baby are the first positive experiences of their lives. Because of the guilt they are harboring, they are often extremely tense during physical examinations. For many this is their first experience with a doctor, hospital, or clinic. Contrary to the general public's belief, many single mothers have had very little sexual experience and what they have had was often negative. Having a vaginal examination is also difficult for them. They certainly do not need to hear the many hurtful cliches that are often reported, eg., "I bet you didn't act this way when you got pregnant."

As her duedate draws near the single woman harbors ambivalent feelings about her impending delivery if she is planning to surrender her baby for adoption. On the one hand she is eager to have the anxieties about labor and delivery behind her and on the other hand she does not want the baby out of her uterus. While she is pregnant, the baby is safe with her at all times and she does not have to face dealing with separating from her baby. This feeling also applies to the woman who is keeping her child because she will then have to face the many struggles of a single parent. Nurses need to be aware that some of the single mothers who are at term have not yet accepted their pregnancy. A simple jubilant comment such as "It won't be long now" or "You'll no doubt keep your next appointment" can open up a whole area of unresolved feelings.

THE SINGLE MOTHER AND CHILDBIRTH EDUCATION

Today many single mothers are attending childbirth preparation classes through the local childbirth education association, public health clinics, or maternity home programs (Fig. 10–1). Many of them choose people other than the baby's father for their labor coaches. Childbirth instructors should address themselves to the "coaches" in their classes rather than the "husbands." The childbirth instructor can make a single mother feel comfortable even in a couples' class.

Even if the mother is planning to surrender her baby for adoption, she should be coached in labor in the same manner as any other woman in labor. Once she has chosen to see the pregnancy to term, it becomes extremely important to her that this baby is healthy and born safely. Large measures of encouragement and praise about the good job she is doing with her breathing exercises and relaxing along with endearments about the fine baby soon to be born really do help the woman to see the pregnancy through positively. This type of experience will also give the woman a feeling of self-esteem. These warm, positive memories which the mother recalls from her labor and delivery often remain with her for many years to come. Hurtful, negative com-

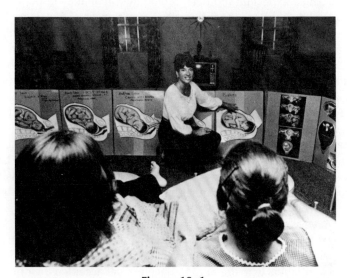

Figure 10–1.

Childbirth education classes in a maternity home offer all necessary information for the single mother to have the positive memories of a prepared delivery.

ments and putdowns which are sometimes offered to the single woman during her labor and delivery are most traumatic to her. These hurtful memories make the difficult time of surrendering the baby even more painful. They also help to eliminate whatever feelings of self-esteem the woman may have begun to realize about herself.

Special Counseling

Counselors work very hard helping the single mother make her OWN decision about how to resolve the pregnancy (Fig. 10-2). It is not up to the nursing personnel to tell the patient how to resolve her pregnancy. Admonition also applies to the parents of the patient and or the baby's father and his parents. Ideal counseling for single mothers should include all the above individuals. The nursing personnel are often not aware of the dynamics of the situation when they meet a single mother and her family. Whatever behaviors or reactions the nursing staff might observe from the expectant mother and/or her parents should be shared with her respective counselors.

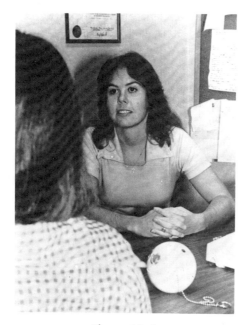

Figure 10-2.

Counselor listens as a client expresses her own decisions.

A nonjudgmental attitude is necessary when dealing with the single mother in all instances. When one is selecting personnel to work with single mothers, it is important to choose a staff that will not offer moralistic judgments above how the woman became pregnant and how she is planning for her child. Before one can appreciate the needs of single mothers, one must understand why they become pregnant in the first place and what they are dealing with. Some reasons that women become pregnant out of wedlock are:

1.   They are seeking love or affection, which they either lack or misinterpret.

2.   Being pregnant puts them in a dependent position and often brings the family closer together.

3.   The pregnancy often replaces the loss of a loved one for whom the woman is still grieving.

4.   Becoming pregnant and producing a life is a source of accomplishment and very often for the particularly deprived woman the pregnancy is the only form of accomplishment she has ever known.

5.   This is the only opportunity some women have to assert their individuality and femininity.

a.   This is particularly true for the girl from a family in which the father is extremely authoritarian and the mother is dominating. Intercourse can be a rebellious act against authoritarian parents.

6.   They have a great lack of knowledge about their own sexuality and sexual function.

a.   Because of this the only way in which these women can communicate with the opposite sex is in a sexual way.

b.   Also because of this lack of knowledge they feel that having intercourse is being loved.

7.   Intercourse is a touching, intimate means of communicating. Women who have never been hugged or cuddled by a parent find that intercourse is a way of fulfilling this need.

8.   In some cases becoming pregnant is a woman's one last effort to hold on to the man she loves.

9.   Some women feel getting pregnant will give them a way to get out of an unpleasant home environment.

DEALING WITH THE SINGLE PREGNANT MOTHER

Once the woman finds herself pregnant she has to deal with many problems. In the first place, for many women, seeing a doctor and having physical examinations are totally new experiences. Having a physician other than the friendly family physician is a tense situation for them. Dealing with the baby's father can also present many problems, expecially if the woman has been abandoned, physically mistreated, or rejected, or is faced with losing the only "love" she has even known. Rejecting her is also a rejection of her unborn child and this too is painful.

Her Parents

She also has to deal with her parents and her immediate family. Very often communication with her family has been strained or nonexistent in the first place. Facing them with this pregnancy is an added strain. Sometimes her parents totally reject their daughter and throw her out of the house. Then, of course, her problems become greater because she needs shelter from the elements and proper nourishment for herself and her unborn child. Other parents offer punishing restrictions on their daughters which increase their shame and guilt. Behavior modification has shown that punishment has never been known to be therapeutic. This is another reason that it is important for the nursing staff not to put forth a punishing attitude when caring for single mothers.

Her Education or Job

The single mother is often dealing with interrupting her education or giving it up entirely. She may also be dealing with losing her job, which may be her only source of income and she needs to face acceptance and/or rejection by her peer group as well. Pregnancies of single mothers are rarely covered by maternity insurance, so she also has to deal with the costs of medical care. We know that many single women have a poor self-image and definitely lack assertiveness. With this type of personality they are not able to face these many social pressures in a healthy way. They simply withdraw and employ defense mechanisms that are often interpreted as arrogant and boastful behavior.

Needs During Labor

It is helpful if the nursing staff asks the single mother during labor if she chooses to see the baby in the delivery room. Situations vary depending on the type of counseling offered from various agencies. For years mothers who surrendered did not see their newborns. Today, we know that every pregnant woman has an image in her mind of what her baby will be like. Such characteristics as sex, physical appearance, who the baby resembles, etc., are included in this image. It tends to become a very detailed picture. One should encourage the woman to talk about this. Many times she will express her feelings about how and why she has this particular fantasy. Interestingly enough, this idealized image never becomes a reality because the fantasy baby is never born.[1]

Psychologists and psychiatrists now believe that it is healthy for the woman to see the child to whom she has given birth. It is very therapeutic for her to see that her child is well formed and healthy. This concept holds true for the mother who gives birth to a child with birth defects or to a stillborn. Seeing her newborn aids her with the separation from her baby and in the acceptance of the pregnancy. Seeing the pregnancy to term, caring for herself during pregnancy, and trying to prepare herself for a safe labor and delivery is the personal gift with which the mother endows her child. She loves to hear all the praises about her baby that any new mother might enjoy hearing: how beautiful, feminine, masculine, tall, short, fat, dimpled, cute, etc. As long as the surrendering mother is not allowed to bond with her infant this can be a positive experience for all involved. If the mother is allowed to see and hold and feed her child on a regular basis, bonding will occur.

A Special Word to Nursing Staff

It might help the obstetrical nursing staff for them to know that even if the mother does not choose to see her baby in the hospital, she has plenty of opportunities to choose to do so until she actually signs surrender papers several weeks later. On the other hand if the mother does see her child, it should be with her counselor who would be best able to handle or help her deal with her feelings. A busy nursery or postpartum nurse usually does not have the time required to stay with the mother when she needs help dealing with her feelings. For those patients who do not have counselors the nurse will possibly have this role. Some single women have a great deal of difficulty accepting their pregnancy because of the circumstances of their conception and also because of the great feelings of guilt they have about having had a sexual relationship and a pregnancy out of wedlock. These women in particular often have a hard time when it comes to the pushing stage of labor. This is particularly true of the women who do become pregnant from having had a one-time sexual experience. They tend to resist the urge to push and

1. Mary Swiger, et al. "Grieving and Unplanned Pregnancy," *Psychiatry*, Feb 1976, pp. 72–80.

show signs of anxiety. When the baby passes through the birth canal, they can no longer resist accepting their pregnancy. Acceptance, patience, compassion, and positive reinforcement on the part of the nursing staff will be helpful at this time.

Talking About the Baby

On the day of delivery the new mother may feel happy and excited. The more counseling she has had the better she will be able to handle this (Fig. 10–3). She will also be much more expressive about her grief and hurt in separating from the baby. She will welcome an opportunity to talk about her child and to accept praise about her accomplishment. Years ago nursing students were taught not to discuss the baby with the woman who was surrendering. Now we know it is more therapeutic if the staff does give the new mother an opportunity to share her feelings if she chooses to do so.

On the first postpartum day the mother may experience a bit of a letdown as with any routine postpartum patient. This is another step toward dealing with the separating from her baby. It is now out of her uterus and she is feeling empty. Every woman who delivers experiences these feelings to some degree. For the surrendering mother this is a more acute experience.

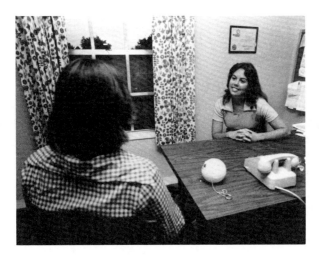

Figure 10–3.

A warm, understanding counselling relationship during pregnancy can help the new mother deal more effectively with her loss.

The mother may name her child if she so chooses. The naming of her child is often a positive sign of the acceptance of her pregnancy. In some areas the baby's first name is used while the child is in foster care. It helps if the nursery staff is aware of this so that the name the mother chooses will be passed on to the caseworker who places the baby in temporary foster care.

Leaving the Hospital

The day that the mother leaves the hospital, usually the second postpartum day, is another step for the mother to deal with in separation. She may well break down and cry and express her feelings of love for her child. This is not a time for the staff to interrogate the mother or to try to talk her into changing her mind about surrendering. This does not indicate that the mother is being forced to surrender or that she does want to change her mind. It is easier for the mother to let go of her child if she can realize her love for it. This too can be a therapeutic experience for her. Some mothers will even show their ambivalence by seeking out a means to keep the child. The length of the hospital stay for the mother will greatly determine that which the nursing staff will observe. The mothers who stay longer than the routine second postpartum day will likely encounter some of these feelings while they are still in the hospital.

For the Mother Who Stays Longer

The third to the fifth postpartum days are particularly crucial. This is the time when their bodies are functioning to complete their role as a mother. Their episiotomy is healing, lactation may occur, and their separation from their baby is most apparent.

The nursing staff's supportive role here is imperative. A nurse may simply ask the patient if she would like company. This is the time to focus on affect with statements such as, "How are you feeling?" or "How do you feel about the baby leaving the hospital today?" or "How do you feel about going home today?" Counselors have worked very hard to teach their clients to express their feelings as they go through this loss. Feelings do not go away. It is therapeutic to express them to someone who is a good listener. This is not an opportunity for one to tell the mother what she should do or to criticize her for her choice.

Today women from cultures that have found surrendering unacceptable in the past are now struggling with new ways to deal with their problem of being pregnant out of wedlock. The pressures their peers put upon them are indeed most painful. Obstetrical supervisors should make a point to instruct their entire staff about the proper way to support these mothers.

Return to Normal With Help

Around the time that the mother is having the first menstrual period following her delivery, she may again experience some of the old feelings of ambivalence. Perhaps she will talk about missing her baby, question her decision, and generally appear depressed. It might be helpful to point out that the hormonal changes after a pregnancy and delivery along with the onset of her menstrual period might well render her more vulnerable at this time. This is usually around the time of her six weeks' checkup. Many times the surrender has not been finalized by the time you see the single mother for this checkup. It takes approximately six to eight weeks for the paperwork to be completed when a woman surrenders her child.

Child-placing agencies do not expect a woman to make a permanent decision about surrendering until several weeks after delivery. Most of the child-placing agencies are licensed by the Child Welfare League of America. Their rules guarantee protection for the woman and her child. If a counselor can see that a woman cannot separate from her baby she will address herself to this problem.

SUMMARY

The single mother deals with many difficult situations during her pregnancy. Perhaps the most difficult is choosing to surrender her baby for adoption. Even though this is her choice, the feeling that she has is very similar to one's reaction to the death of a loved one. She needs to get in touch with this grief process. It takes approximately six weeks for intensive grieving to take place, although a sense of loss continues for a long period of time thereafter.

BIBLIOGRAPHY

Badger E, Burns D, Rhoads B: Education for Adolescent Mothers in a Hospital Setting, *American Journal of Public Health,* May 1976.

Frye BA, Barham B: Reaching Out to Pregnant Adolescents, *American Journal of Nursing,* Sep 1975.

Personal communication with Dr. R. Good, Psychiatrist–Obstetrician, School of Medicine, University of Miami, 1977.

Klerman L: Adolescent Pregnancy: The Need for New Policies and New Programs, *Journal of School Health,* May 1975.

Lindeman E: "Symptomatology and Management of Acute Grief," *American Journal of Psychiatry,* Sep 1944, pp. 141–48.

Schwartz BA: Rock and 'Bye Baby *JOGN,* Sep/Oct 1975.

Smith EW: The Role of the Grandmother in Adolescent Pregnancy and Parenting, *Journal of School Health,* May 1975.

Taylor D: A New Way to Teach Teens About Contraceptives, *American Journal of Maternal and Child Nursing,* Nov/Dec 1976.

Vincent CE: *Unwed Mothers* (Glencoe, Ill: Free Press, 1961).

Chapter 11

Assisting Parents of High-Risk Infants

MARGARET ZACHA TAYLOR, RN, MNEd

The development of medical and nursing care for infants who are premature or ill at birth has focused on their physiological needs. Little concern has been shown for the needs of the families involved. In the fifties and sixties all high-risk infants were separated from their parents at birth and were immediately placed in premature nurseries. Because the infant was at increased risk of infection in addition to the already existing problems, the parents were not allowed to touch their infant throughout the neonate's entire hospitalization. They could only view their infant through the glass window in the nursery. On the day of discharge the baby was removed from the premature nursery and given to the parents to feed and dress for the first time.

NEW TRENDS IN NEONATAL CARE

In the late sixties and early seventies great advances were made in the care of these "high-risk infants," but the new treatment modalities necessitated sophisticated equipment and more technical skills. Because these new procedures and equipment required specially trained staff, the new neonatal units were expensive to operate, and their cost was beyond the capabilities of most local hospitals. Therefore, the majority of states developed a system of regional nurseries to which high-risk infants could be transferred. This regionalization often necessitates transferring infants away from the community in which they were born. In Florida, one of the first states to develop this system of regional neonatal nurseries, an infant can be transferred a distance of more than 150 miles. The care given to high-risk infants in these special neonatal units is increasing their survival rate and allowing them to develop with a higher potential for wellness than was previously possible.

Problems for Parents

Unfortunately, regional nurseries provide additional problems for families who want to visit their infants and to monitor closely infant progress. One of these problems is financial. Long-distance telephone calls, trips to the neonatal regional center, and the cost of having an infant in the neonatal unit can amount to considerable expense for the parents. Also, focus on the physiological needs of the infant has tended to bring about a health care delivery system that has increased the psychological distance between high-risk infants and their parents. Inadequate though the care was in local hospitals, at least parents could regularly view their infants.

Response to Parental Needs

Demand by parents for greater participation in the care of their infants and clinical recognition of the value of parental contact has led some regional nurseries to open their doors to the parents. At first this was done only on a trial basis. When no increase in infection was noted, a policy of regular contact between parents and their infants was adopted. But, although the parents are allowed in the nursery, there is little nursing care directed at meeting their needs. The health care team still sees the infant as a separate entity and not in the context of the relationship between parents and child. Parents are judged by what they do to meet the physiological needs of the infant, not by how satisfactorily they are developing their role as parents. The nursing staff allows the parents to see and touch the infant, and there is an explanation of what care is being given and the reasons for the care, but nursing notes in neonatal units do not discuss the parents and their response to the infant or the infant's response to the parents. Often there is not even a record of the parents visiting the infant. This lack of documentation is vital when the only documented evidence of future parenting difficulties is visiting or telephoning by parents concerning their infant five or more times within a two-week period.[1]

High-Risk Parents

Studies done in the sixties indicate that parents of high-risk infants have problems in maintaining adequate parenting. Studies done in 1967 and 1968 indicate that a high percentage of children who do not thrive without a known physiological basis[2] and children who are abused[3] have a common history of being ill at birth or being premature. Green and Solnit[4] noted that a syndrome they coined, "the vulnerable child syndrome," develops when infants or children live who had been expected to die. The parents of such children are overly anxious about the health of these children and find it difficult to accept the assurance of health team members that their children are developing normally. Barnett in 1970[5] studied interactional deprivation as a source of mothering problems and documented three differences between mothers who were separated from their newborns at birth and mothers who were not separated. The three differences in the separated mothers were: 1) less commitment or attachment to the infant, 2) less confidence in their mothering abilities, and 3) less ability to establish an efficient care-taking regimen.

Even with the evidence provided in these studies, nursing staff members of neonatal units have not focused on the needs of parents of high-risk infants to develop their parenting role. Indeed, it seems that the lack of concern for parental needs is common throughout the parent–child health area. However, because studies indicate that parents of high-risk infants are themselves at risk for developing parenting skills, and because the methods developed for delivering health care to high-risk infants make it difficult for these parents to develop these skills, it is especially important that the nursing goals be expanded to include helping such parents develop their parenting skills.

1.   A. Fanaroff, J. Kennell, and M. Klaus, "Follow-up Care of Low Birth Weight Infants: The Predictive Value of Maternal Visiting Patterns," *Pediatrics,* 1972, p. 287.

2.   E. Shaheed, D. Alexander, J. Truskowsky, and G. Barbero, "Failure to Thrive—a Retrospective Profile," *Clinical Pediatrics,* 1968, p. 255.

3.   E. Elmer and G. Gregg, "Developmental Characteristics of Abused Children," *Pediatrics,* 1964, p. 58.

4.   Morris Green, and Albert J. Solnit, "Reactions to the Threatened Loss of a Child: A Vulnerable Child Syndrome," *Pediatrics,* 1964, p. 58.

5.   C. Barnett, P. Leiderman, R. Brobstein, and M. Klaus, "Neonatal Separation," *Pediatrics,* 1970, p. 197.

MOTHER-INFANT RELATIONSHIPS

Although Keirnon and Scoloveno[6] state that parenting functions can be considered human functions and need not be separated into mothering and fathering, the remainder of this chapter will apply theory relating only to the development of mothering. By applying this theory, the nurse should be able to assist a grieving mother of a high-risk infant in becoming a mother who can achieve satisfactions in implementing her mothering role in relation to her new infant.

Infant Bonding

Rubin[7] in a recent article noted that there are three mutually dependent aspects of the "binding-in" process that occur after delivery. These are identification, claiming, and polarization. Rubin prefers the term *binding-in attachment* or *bonding* because it describes the formative phases of the maternal–child relationship as a process, rather than a state.

Identification
Identification involves the direct verification of the infant based on sex, size, and condition. A mother needs to know the child's condition before she can react to or interact with her infant.

Claiming
Claiming refers to such activities as inclusion of the infant in a social sphere of those persons the mother claims as her own and who, in turn, claim her. One such activity occurs when the mother states in detail that the infant has a "nose like Uncle Jim, hair like his brother, Larry, and ears like Cousin John."

Polarization
Polarization is the process of separation of the mother from the infant. For a mother of a normal-term infant this process of binding-in takes one to three months.

6.   Barbara Kierman, and Mary Ann Scoloveno, "Fathering," *Nursing Clinics of North America,* 1977, p. 481.
7.   Reva Rubin, "Binding-In In the Post Partum Period," *American Journal of Maternal Child Nursing, May/Jun* 1977, p. 67.

Mothers and Term Infants

Studies indicate certain activities allow mothers of normal-term babies to achieve a positive relationship with their infants. Holding her infant right after birth gives the mother a chance to begin the identifying and claiming activities so important in binding-in. Furthermore, Rubin states:

> Externalization seems to be a singularly important aspect of polarization to the new mother. At delivery the experience of feeling the baby outside her body, on the surface of her body, across her abdomen or in her arms is particularly meaningful. A woman who has not had this experience does not seem to feel that she has given birth to a child or that she has been given a child.[8]

Maternal attachment, or bonding, is the term that Klaus uses in describing the unique relationship between the mother and her infant, a relationship that is specific and endures through time. Klaus believes that there may be an optimal time for this relationship to begin, which may be in the first hour of life.[9] In the first hour after delivery, mothers need to see, touch, hold, fondle, and suckle their infants. If given the opportunity, mothers will continue to observe, touch, hold, and fondle their infants for long periods of time, thus building the relationship between them. They will often hold their infants in an "en face" position, which fosters mother–child interactions. The "en face" position as defined by Klaus occurs when the mother's face is rotated so that her eyes and those of the infant meet fully in the same vertical plane. Klaus thinks there are several activities that form the basis for interactions between the mother and the infant, and, therefore, the basis for the development of maternal–child bonding.[10] These occur together and interlock, but for reasons of clarity, the activities noted will be mentioned separately and sequentially.

Klaus: Bonding Sequence for Mother

The mother initiates interactions with the infant by the following means:

Touch. Rubin's description[11] of the maternal touch is clearly presented and readily observed as the mother begins to relate to her newborn. The mother

8. *Ibid.,* p. 73.
9. Marshall Klaus, et al, "Maternal Attachment: Importance of the First Few Days Postpartum," *New England Journal of Medicine,* 1972, p. 460.
10. Marshall Klaus, and J. Kennell, *Maternal–Infant Bonding,* (St. Louis: C. V. Mosby Co, 1976, p. 67–82.
11. Reva Rubin, "Maternal Touch," *Nursing Outlook,* 1963, p. 828.

begins with fingertips and moves in a definite pattern toward embracing the infant in her arms.

Eye-to-eye contact. Mothers are anxious to see their newborns' eyes open and need to achieve eye-to-eye contact. They are concerned if their newborns never open their eyes. Also, as previously mentioned, the mothers need to look into their infants' eyes from an "en face" position.

Speaking in a high-pitched voice. Brazelton reports that a neonate is more alert and attentive to a female voice than a low-pitched male voice. Therefore, talking in the high-pitched voice that mothers readily use for conversation with their newborns fits into the infant's sensitive auditory perception pattern.

Entrainment or response to speech pattern. When the mother speaks to her newborn, the baby moves in time with the structure of her speech. When the speaker pauses for breath or accents a syllable, the infant almost imperceptibly raises an eyebrow or lowers a foot. The infant, from the beginning, is conditioned to having movements synchronized with adult speech patterns.

Time Giver. Infants after birth are in a state of disequilibrium. Rhythms such as the mother's heartbeat, patterns of sleeping and waking, patterns of work and rest, which influenced them in intrauterine life are gone. The mother through her establishment of a routine in the early days after delivery assists the neonate in reestablishing his/her rhythm.

Klaus: Bonding Sequence for Infant
The infant also contributes to the mother–child interactions. Klaus mentions the following four ways in which the infant contributes to the interaction pattern or initiates the interactions between himself/herself and the mother.

Eye-to-eye contact. The infant looks at the mother's face. It is interesting to note that infants can focus best at a distance of 12 inches. This is the approximate distance in the breast-feeding position.

Infant cry. Crying by the baby when he or she becomes uncomfortable for any reason will pull the mother to her infant.

Hormones. The infant, through the breast-feeding process, initiates the secretion of the maternal hormones oxytocin and prolactin. In studies noted by Klaus, prolactin, which is increased in the mother during nursing as well as while holding and fondling the infant, has been identified as a "love" hormone in birds. It may be that this hormone assists in the establishment of positive relationships between the mother and her infant (see footnote 4).

Entrainment. Entrainment is also an important area in which the infant can contribute to the mother–child relationship. It is the infant's response to the mother's speech pattern that allows the mother to feel that communication, the basis of any relationship, is occurring.

Mothering Tasks

In addition to the need for the preceding elements to provide the opportunity for bonding or binding-in to occur, the mother also needs to gain confidence in her ability to comfort, feed, and care for her infant. The first task of mothering is to develop skill in feeding the infant.[12] The first feeding experience is very important for the mother as she needs success in accomplishing this task if she is to continue to progress toward feeling good about her mothering abilities. Mothers will then move to developing skill at comforting their infants, changing diapers, bathing their babies, and all the other tasks of mothering.

Mothers and High-Risk Infants

If the components identified by Klaus as maternal–child bonding and by Rubin as binding-in are necessary for the mother to establish her mothering role, nurses especially need to encourage these interactions between mothers and their high-risk infants. Providing for these interactions is not now part of the routine care given to mothers of high-risk infants. Consider a case in which a mother delivers a three-pound infant. She does not have the opportunity to hold her infant after delivery. The baby is often immediately transferred to another facility that has a neonatal intensive care unit. Usually the mother will be given the opportunity to view the infant for a short time, but the infant is in an incubator and, often, in an oxygen hood. There is little opportunity to assist the mother in the early tasks of identification, claiming, and polarization because her contact with the infant is so limited. Also, the components necessary for maternal bonding are not possible when the mother and infant are separated.

Besides this inability to provide the opportunity for binding-in and maternal bonding, nurses often spend little time with the mothers of high-risk infants and give them only minimal care. The lack of contact with the mothers may

12.   Reva Rubin, "Basic Maternal Behavior," *Nursing Outlook,* 1961, p. 683.

be due to insufficient knowledge about the needs of the mother of a high-risk infant. Families also isolate these parents. Family and friends hesitate to congratulate the mother on the birth of a three-pound infant whose condition is unstable. Health team members are often pessimistic about the infant's chance for survival. They may voice their concern to the parents or may avoid discussions with the parents. Health team members need to be as hopeful as the infant's condition permits. "If a mother is to mother her child adequately throughout the rest of his childhood, she must begin building a firm and close tie with him at birth. Pessimistic remarks during the first hours of life cause a premature infant's mother to hold back, stifling this bond at its inception, and to embark on the process of anticipatory grief."[13]

Tasks

Health team members have certain tasks to accomplish as they work with parents of high-risk infants.

1. These mothers must work through their grief over the loss of their idealized infant and learn to accept their newborn. The mother needs to discuss her feelings about the infant and her reactions toward seeing the baby.[14]

2. This mother must begin to resolve her guilt feelings about producing a small or ill infant. This guilt often immobilizes the mother, preventing her from asking questions about her child as well as establishing a relationship with her/him. Being able to verbalize her feelings and obtaining some explanation of the causes of the infant's condition is an important step toward resolving these feelings.[15]

3. The mother needs to regain self-esteem. She has a sense of failure when she delivers a small infant or one who is ill at birth; she has failed in her maternal role.[16] This lack of self-esteem may be manifested by discussion of successes as well as failures. In a small study this author conducted with mothers of high-risk infants, each subject first discussed in great depth all her achievements in her life; then she asked questions about why the infant had come early and expressed concern over her maternal abilities.

4. The mother needs to have ongoing contact with her infant and needs to have roles that she can play in the care. Nursing staff need to focus on how the infant and mother relate to each other and share these observations with

13.   Klaus and Kennell, op. cit., p. 124.
14.   Bertrand Cramer, "A Mother's Reaction to the Birth of a Premature Baby" in Klaus and Kennell, op. cit., p. 161.
15.   Ibid. p. 158.
16.   Ibid.

the mother. This sharing with the mother will assist her in developing her relationship with the infant. Having one or more definite tasks that she can do is also very important. This task can be talking with the infant and touching his or her hand or head for five minutes four times a day as well as bathing or feeding the infant. Mothers should be given a task that is "their task" because this will increase self-esteem and assist in the maternal bonding. Mothers respond well to this approach as long as they are given support while they begin to implement their role (Figure 11–1).

5. The mother will need to know how to care for her infant after discharge. If the previous tasks have been accomplished, the mother will have gained a knowledge of the infant's need and responses and will have established a relationship with her infant. Additional support is needed, of course, in preparing for discharge of the infant and transferring the complete care to the mother.

STANDARDS OF CARE

Standards of care are the basis of quality nursing care (Fig. 11–2) and are as needed in the neonatal units as in any nursing care unit. The special standards of care for neonatal nursing should encompass biopsychosocial needs of mothers of high-risk infants and should give guidelines for assessing the mother's ability to incorporate the components of maternal–child bonding or binding-in. Since there appears to be a lack of standards other than those dealing with maternal or infant physical recovery, the following are proposed using the ANA Guidelines as a resource for structure (Fig. 11–3).

For a complete explanation of standard writing and criteria formation, the reader is referred to Guidelines for Review of Nursing Care at the Local Level published by the American Nurses' Association.[17] These standards reflect how the nursing staff should be assisting the mother in establishing an attachment to her infant and serve as a guide for the clinical data that should be recorded in the nursing notes. These proposed standards have not yet been tested nor are they intended to be adopted as the only standards for this population. Alterations of the criteria and the time frame within which they are to be met may be needed. When clinical data on these criteria become available from nursing notes, then these should be altered as appropriate. They are offered

17. ———,Guidelines for Review of Nursing Care at the Local Level (Kansas City, Mo: The American Nurses Association).

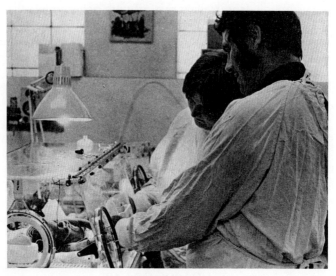

Figure 11–1.

In perinatal centers, parents are encouraged to join in the care of their infants. (From Mecca Cranley, "When a High-Risk Infant Is Born," *American Journal of Nursing,* Oct. 1975. Reprinted with permission of author and American Journal of Nursing.)

Figure 11–2.

Criteria, standards, and norms—definitions.*

Criteria: A criterion (or criterion variable or parameter) is the value-free name of a variable believed or known to be a relevant indicator of the quality of patient care (medical care or nursing care).

Standard: A standard is the desired and achievable level (or range) of performance corresponding with a criterion (or criterion variable or parameter) against which actual performance is compared.

Norm: A norm is the current level or range of performance corresponding with a criterion (or criterion variable or parameter) and is determined by descriptive study of "the here and now" in a given population, region, institution, group, and so forth.

*From Doris Bloch, "Criteria, Standards and Norms—Crucial Terms in Quality Assurance" *Journal of Nursing Administration* Sept 1977, p. 22, 26. (Reprinted with permission of Journal of Nursing Administration.)

Figure 11-3.

Criteria for nursing care—maternal–infant relationship.

Target Population: Management of a woman who delivered a preterm infant

Variables: 1. Vaginal delivery
2. First preterm infant
3. Second infant
4. 20–30 years of age

Criteria Subset	Screening Criteria	Critical Time	Standard	Exception	Documentation
The mother will identify her feelings and reactions regarding the early labor experience	The woman will: 1. Describe what happened during pregnancy and before labor	Before discharge from hospital	100%	None	John Kennell and Marshall Klaus, "Caring for Parents of a Premature or Sick Infant," *Maternal-Infant Bonding* (St. Louis: C. V. Mosby Company, 1976) p. 99.
	2. Discuss what she would have done if she could do things over again	Before discharge from hospital	100%	None	Ann Clark and Dyanne Alfonso, *Childbearing: A Nursing Perspective* (Philadelphia: F. A. Davis Company, 1976), p. 458.
	3. Discuss the physiological reasons for the early labor	Before discharge from hospital	100%	None	Bertrand Cramer "A Mother's Reactions to the Birth of a Premature Infant," *Maternal-Infant Bonding* (St. Louis: C. V. Mosby Company, 1976), p. 156.
	4. Discuss her concerns regarding the laboring experience: 1. Her expectations 2. Her responses	Before discharge from hospital	100%	None	

Figure 11-3. (Continued)

Criteria Subset	Screening Criteria	Critical Time	Standard	Exception	Documentation
The mother will identify the characteristics of the infant	The woman will:				
	1. Discuss her ideas of what infant will be like	Before first visit of infant	100%	None	Ibid.
	2. Contrast new infant's characteristics with past term infant	By third visit to nursery	100%	If infant's condition is unstable	Kennell and Klaus, loc. cit.
	3. Discuss reasons for infant's treatments	Before third visit to nursery	100%	Same as above	Reva Rubin, "Binding-in in the Postpartum Period," *Maternal-Child Nursing*, **6:2** (Summer 1977), p. 67.
	4. Begin to identify who child is like	By third visit to nursery	100%	Same as above	
	5. Name her infant	By third visit to nursery	100%	None	
	6. Discuss her concerns regarding infant's future	By third visit to nursery	100%	If infant's condition is unstable	
The mother will identify her role in the infant's care	The woman will:				
	1. Identify areas and ways she can interact with infant	By third visit to nursery	100%	Same as above	Ibid.
	2. Seek eye-to-eye contact with infant with the staff's assistance	By third visit to nursery	100%	Same as above	
	3. Discuss one way the infant reacts to her voice or touch	By third visit to nursery	100%	Same as above	

The mother will implement her role in the infant's care				
The woman will:				
1. Call or visit the nursery every day or every other day	By the end of the first week of the infant's life	100%	None	A. Fanaroff, J. Kennell, and M. Klaus, "Follow-up of Low Birth-weight-infants: The Predictive Value of Maternal Visiting Patterns," *Pediatrics*, **49:**278, 1972.
2. Touch and talk to infant without assistance from staff	By the end of the second week of the infant's life	100%	None	Cramer, op. cit. Kennell and Klaus, op. cit.
3. Actively seek eye-to-eye contact with infant without assistance from staff	By the end of the second week of the infant's life	100%	None	Rubin, op. cit. Reva Rubin, "Maternal Touch," *Nursing Outlook*, **11:**11 (November 1963) p. 828.
4. Discuss the infant's reactions to her	By the end of the second week of the infant's life	100%	None	
5. Continue to seek verification of the infant's condition	By the end of the second week of the infant's life			
6. Discuss freely who the infant looks like and acts like	By the end of the first week of the infant's life	100%	None	
7. Assist in bathing the infant	By the end of the second week of the infant's life	100%	If infant's condition is unstable	
8. Hold infant close in her arms	Within four days when this is possible	100%	None	
9. Feeds infant	Within four days when this is possible	100%	None	
10. Expresses satisfaction from holding and feeding infant	Within one week when this is possible	100%	None	

184

Figure 11-3. (Continued)

Criteria Subset	Screening Criteria	Critical Time	Standard	Exception	Documentation
The mother will involve significant others in the establishment of affectional bonds to infant	The woman will:				Kennell and Klaus, op. cit. Cramer, op. cit.
	1. Include father in discussions about the infant's condition	By the second visit to infant in nursery	100%	No father figure available	
	2. Encourage father to visit infant with or without her	By second visit to nursery	100%	Same as above	
	3. Encourage father to touch and/or hold infant	By second visit to nursery	100%	Same as above	
	4. Take pictures of infant or encourage siblings and grandparents to visit nursery and see infant	By second week of infant's life	100%	None	
	5. Discuss reactions of friends to infant's birth, condition, and/or future	One week before discharge	100%	If infant is discharged within one week of birth then needs to occur two days prior to discharge	
	6. Discuss plans for care of infant discharge: acceptance into family, physical care aspects, affectional needs and medical care	One week before discharge	100%	Same as above	

here as one attempt to translate the theory of supporting mothers of high-risk infants into a practicable guideline for evaluating nursing care.

SUMMARY

The survival of high-risk neonates has greatly improved in the past decade because of increased technology and the availability of regional centers that provide for the special needs of these babies. The very care that improves chances for neonatal survival imposes special problems for the parents of the high-risk infant.

Special nursing effort must be made to assist the parents of these problem babies to achieve the tasks vital to their assuming the active role of parent to their own child. One approach to developing nursing care for these parents is to try to identify the standard of care that would have to be met if the parenting sense is to emerge.

BIBLIOGRAPHY

Anderson GC: The Mother and Her Newborn: Mutual Care Givers, *JOGN*, Sept/Oct 1977.

Barnett C et al: Neonatal Separation: The Maternal Side of the Interactional Deprivation, *Pediatrics* **45**:197, 205, 1970.

Berger GS et al, The Evaluation of Regionalized Perinatal Health, *American Journal Obstetrics and Gynecology*, Aug 1, 1976.

Carron RB: The Development of Maternal Touch During Early Mother–Infant Interaction, *JOGN* **6**:2, Mar/Apr 1977.

Cranley MS: When a High Risk Infant Is Born, *American Journal of Nursing* **75**:10, Oct 1975.

Cureton M (Premature and High Risk Infant Assn., P. O. Box A-3083, Peoria, Ill): Her Ten Days in September Had to Have a Meaning, *American Journal of Nursing* **76**:8, Aug 1976.

Eches S: The Significance of Increased Early Contact Between Mother and Newborn Infant *JOGN* **3**:4, Jul/Aug 1974.

Gluck L et al: Neonatal Intensive Care Units in Community Hospitals and Remote Areas, *Clinical Perinatology* **3**:10, Sep 1976.

Harrison LK: Making a Good Thing Better: Regionalization of Neonatal Intensive Care Units, *JOGN* **4**:3, May/Jun 1975.

Hawes WE, Hodgman J: High Risk Perinatal Care in California, *Western Journal of Medicine* **124**:1, Jan 1976.

Hurd JM: Assessing Maternal Attachment: The First Step Toward Preventing Child Abuse, *JOGN* **4**:4, Jul/Aug 1975.

Johnson SH, Grubbs JP: The Premature Infants' Reflex Behavior. Effects on Maternal–Child Relationship, *JOGN* **4**:3, May/Jun 1975.

Kennedy J: The High Risk Maternal–Infant Acquaintance Process, *NURS Clin of N. America* **8**:549–56, 1973.

Klaus M, Kennell JH: Mother Separation from Their Newborn Infants, *Pediatric Clinics of North America,* Nov 1970.

Merkatz IR, Johnson KG: Regionalization of Perinatal Care for the United States, *Clinical Perinatology* **3**:10, Sep 1976.

Neligan GA et al: *Born Too Soon or Born Too Small.* Philadelphia, J. B. Lippincott, 1976.

Penfold KM: Supporting Mother Love, American Journal of Nursing **74**:3, Mar 1974.

Schneider JM, Graves SN: Regionalized OB/GYN Care in Wisconsin *Contemporary OB/GYN* **3**:3, Mar 1974.

Shearer MH: The Effects of Regionalization of Perinatal Care on Hospital Services for Normal Childbirth, *Birth and the Family Journal* **4**:4, Winter 1977.

Slade C et al: Working with Parents of High Risk Newborns, *JOGN* **6**:2, Mar/Apr 1977.

Stern L: Prematurity As a Factor in Child Abuse, *Hospital Practice* **8**:5, May 1973.

PART FOUR

CHANGE AND THE FUTURE

This part is designed to explore the possibilities for the future of childbirth education. With the use of the diagrammatic organizational model developed by Bartlett and Kayser, the present and future are compared in terms of structural variables. Because the main concept of futurology is that change is always with us, the relevance of change and resistance to change is described in relation to childbirth education and the larger system within which it exists.

Several alternatives are presented as the basis for future developments in practice settings for childbirth—the homelike birthing room, the family hospital, and the childbearing center. These developments are presented to expand nursing perception of childbirth beyond the stereotyped "obstetrical unit," and to provide reasonable compromises for those parents who would risk danger or death rather than accept the conditions available in traditional maternity settings.

Chapter 12

Options for the Future

Scientists have already predicted what life will probably be like in the year 2000. It is no secret that if humankind is to survive, a different kind of life-style will have to emerge. Exactly what that will be is still a bit hazy at this time. And, so it is in the field of childbirth education. There is no doubt that care of expectant and new families will be different, but the question remains: Where do we go from here? There is no clearcut answer because there are several possible options opening up now. Which option the established medical community will elect remains to be seen. But, the parents of this society are making their desires well known. Family-centered care is at the base of every option. Participative obstetrics and cooperative parenting are real, the desire for them is being expressed, and the structure in which they can occur can take several forms.

CHANGE FOR THE FUTURE

One might ask why, if the consumers of the services are making their requirements clearly known, does the service not meet their needs? There are two answers: 1) the environment in which the service is offered—the traditional hospital setting—and 2) the fear of the unknown that is generated

189

when any change in an accepted ritual is suggested. Of course, these are not the reasons publicly espoused. The public reasons usually center around patient safety and cost containment. However, when one considers that the health care industry is one of the largest dollar volume businesses in the country and begins to apply the models of business and industry to the management of health care institutions, then through this different frame of reference it becomes easier to understand the phenomenon.

A Model for Change

As professional change agents in industry, Bartlett and Kayser developed a model for describing and dissecting the organization.[1] Within the forces external to the organization that govern its basic values and goals, there function several subsystems that lead to the achievement or nonachievement of the formal goals of the organizations. By comparing the behavioral consequences with the formal organizational goals, an observer can learn if the organization is effectively and efficiently doing what it is intended to do (Fig. 12–1).

External Factors

Plugging childbirth education movement into the Bartlett–Kayser model helps to explain the present dilemma. Using as a prototype of the traditional hospital an urban institution of 200 beds, consider the influence of the external factors (Fig. 12–2).

Social conditions. These have changed. Parents are questioning whether to have children as their parents did, often limiting their families to one or two. People in general have come to question the value of psychological as well as physical health and seek caregivers who can provide both.

Environmental changes. There is greater awareness of the ecosystem that includes Homo sapiens. People are questioning many commonplace things in their environment and the threat that they pose to present and future life. This includes technological advances in medical science.

Cultural changes. Values of dignity and human worth are being emphasized over property and the physical world.

1. Alton C. Bartlett, and Thomas A. Kayser, Eds, *Changing Organizational Behavior* (Englewood Cliffs, NJ: Prentice-Hall, 1973), pp. 4–14.

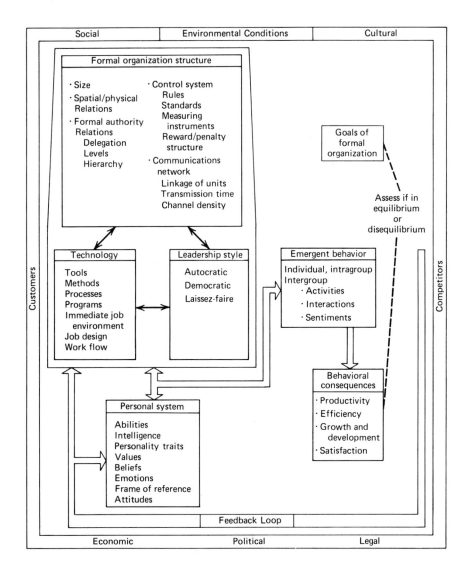

Figure 12–1.

The Bartlett–Kayser Model—an organization from a "change agent's" frame of reference.

191

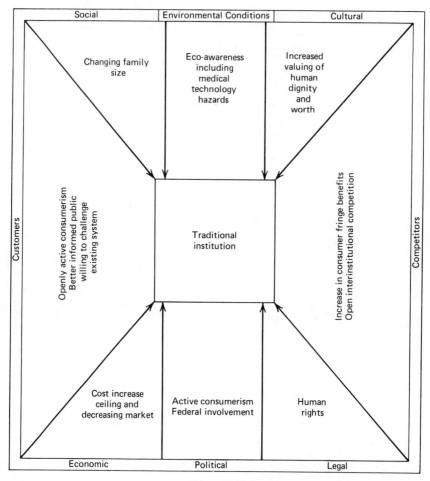

Figure 12–2.

External forces impinging on traditional institutions. (Adapted from Bartlett AC, Kayser TA: *Changing Organizational Behavior:* Englewood Cliffs, N.J., Prentice-Hall, 1973, p. 6. Adapted by permission.)

Legal changes. The rapid changes in constitutional law in the past 20 years have opened new vistas. The entire question of right versus privilege has considerable weight in the childbirth education movement.

Political changes. The burgeoning of active consumerism has influenced the determinations of the elected representatives. The increasing role of the

Federal government in the health care industry will undoubtedly influence development.

Economic changes. With a 9% ceiling increase on the cost of health care, the institutions are being forced to look at cost effective care. Maternity care has historically been one of the most expensive services that hospitals offer. Many institutions have closed down these services to economize. Others are looking at the services very closely for future direction.

Competitors. In a free enterprise economy, competition has always been an important factor. It has been difficult for hospitals to admit that they are in competition. However, when it is obvious that the market of expectant couples is shrinking, then the agencies offering them services are definitely in competition; each trying to lure all paying customers from the other by offering a variety of nonessential fringe benefits that are designed to appeal to the consumer. Some institutions have developed entire family-centered programs in an attempt to meet the consumer demand by providing a service not available with their competitors.

Consumers. Of all the forces external to the institutions, consumers have made the most sustained effort to try to influence the health care institutions to provide family-centered care including childbirth education. Capitalizing on the economic, political, and legal forces impinging on the hospitals, consumers have consistently tried to influence the traditional hospital establishment to bring about the changes that would allow family-centered care. Their efforts have met with varying degrees of success. In the early 1950s, the external forces lacked the combined power of the external forces of the 1970s. Many institutions have moved toward family-centered care, at least in name, because of the combined influence of the extrainstitutional pressures beyond their control. However, it was never the intent of those who supported family-centered care that the philosophy be superimposed on a system that is in reality unchanged except for a few functional concessions selected because they represent little or no increase in cost.

The Formal Organization Structure

The actual formal organizational system will probably have the most far-reaching influence on how an idea or philosophy is actually carried out in that agency. The system consists of three distinct elements: the formal structure, the leadership style, and the technology available to achieve the organization's goals. Many traditionally conceived hospitals offering maternity services tend to be large, with the result that they can absorb the cost of this service; tend to be built for the convenience of the physicians and sometimes the nurses who will work in them; tend to be internally structured along the lines of a pyramid with each level of worker reporting to a higher level with the ultimate responsibility belonging to the administrator, who reports to a board of trustees or directors. The only fallacy in this model is that the hospital is the only hierarchical structure in which the lower levels of the hierarchy are subject to the intervening authority of an external force—the physician. Controls tend to be by rules subject to reward and punishment. And, communications tend to be downward and frequently in writing. The overall impression is dehumanizing for the workers in the system, who have little or no power and who survive or perish on their ability to uphold the system. Within this kind of formal structure, the leadership style that pervades is basically autocratic both from the formal structure and from the external intervening force. There are usually vast amounts of technological equipment and methods available and used to justify its existence.

When family-centered care is superimposed on this kind of system, the results are usually less than desirable. In order for family-centered care to be truly effective, the formal system needs changing so that the focus is shifted from the workers to the consumers. In an ideal setting for family-centered care, the spatial relationships would be family-oriented in that provisions are made to meet the basic needs of the family members as well as the client, or rather the family is perceived as the client instead of the single person who receives the main service. Formal authority relations would include the family in planning and feedback, with the presence and advice of the physician and the nurse being that of expert resource. In this system, the rewards could be based on the achievement and evaluation of client-care objectives. And, the communication system would involve upward, downward, and lateral communication with the opportunity for all participants to contribute. The leadership style in this setting would be participative. The technology available would be used when needed in the opinion of the experts and by mutual agreement (Fig. 12–3).

Personal Systems

The preceding projection is, of course, fantasy. The reason it does not now exist is that the personal systems of those key people in the organizations may be at odds with the personal systems of the clients (Fig. 12–4). For example, those characteristics that make it possible for a physician to survive and graduate from medical school and those characteristics that make it possible for a nurse to survive in a hospital hierarchy may be exactly those things that will be in conflict with the goals of parents who are seeking family-centered care in which they will be able to have some say about that care.

Chris Argyris, in discussing organizational effectiveness, identifies interper-

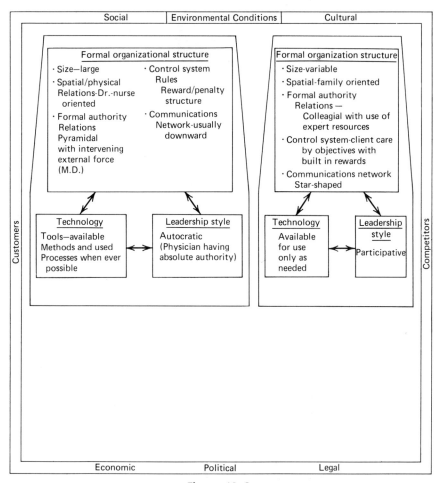

Figure 12–3.

Formal system—real and ideal. (Adapted from Bartlett AC, Kayser TA: *Changing Organizational Behavior.* Englewood Cliffs, N.J., Prentice-Hall, 1973, p. 6. Adapted by permission.)

sonal competence as an important element.[2] The components in interpersonal competence include risk-taking, willingness to own up, and giving and receiving descriptive, nonevaluative feedback. For many health professionals, these characteristics have been systematically eliminated from their daily repertoire—in part because of fear of personal reprisal in the system and in

2.   Chris Argyris, *Interpersonal Competence and Organizational Effectiveness* (Homewood, Ill: The Dorsey Press, 1962).

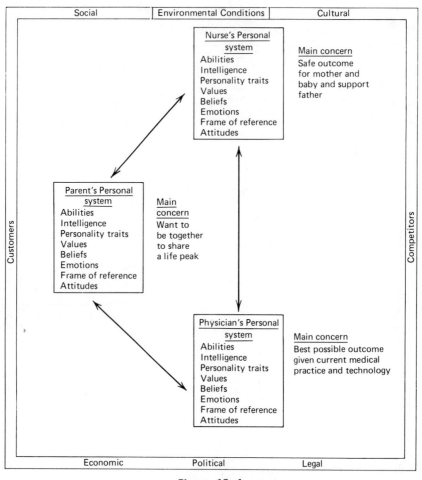

Figure 12–4.

Personal systems—potential conflict. (Adapted from Bartlett AC, Kayser TA: *Changing Organizational Behavior*. Englewood Cliffs, N.J., Prentice-Hall, 1973, p. 6. Adapted by permission.)

part because of fear of litigation should fallibility be admitted. Therefore, personal systems often reflect the survival need of self-protection that isolates the care-givers from the recipients (Fig. 12–4).

Emergent Behavior
One outcome of the barriers in the traditional hospital structure is what Bartlett calls emergent behavior, that is unusual or difficult-to-explain behav-

ior of individuals or groups.[3] The emergent behavior seen in the childbirth education movement is the increasing number of documented home deliveries. Most professionals react with horror at this development, citing many examples of "nick of time" medical intervention that saved the life of a mother or baby in the hospital. How, they ask, can parents take such a chance? The answer is that for some parents, the chance of an out-of-control emergency with the possibility of a tragic outcome is worth the risk when compared with the definite alternative of traditional hospital care, which limits who can be present, what technology will be used, and what decisions the parents can make about the process they are experiencing. The parents who choose a home delivery may be considering economic factors as well. Before they are condemned completely, perhaps the alternatives need to be made available that will meet the parents' needs.

Future Orientation

The hospitals that will be able to meet parents' needs in the year 2000 are future-oriented today. The prototype used to satirize traditional hospital care would be described by Lippitt as a static organization[4] (Fig. 12–5). Many large organizations do fall into this category. They are characterized by a low level of job satisfaction and a high rate of employee turnover. This is characteristic of many hospitals as well. The turning point for the future will be the professional nurses who recognize the importance of understanding and applying organizational management theory to hospital nursing practice and can wield enough power in the hospital system to bring about change. Nursing represents the largest percentage of the work force in the hospital and yet has historically had little influence until the present. Nurses in leadership positions who are well educated are becoming more and more able to direct for the future. However, the education must include the ability to deal with change and the resistance engendered when change is proposed. For the fear of change is the biggest ally of the status quo.

3. Bartlett and Kayser, op. cit. p. 5.
4. Gordon L. Lippitt, "Hospital Organization in the Post Industrial Society" Hospital Progress, July 1973.

Figure 12–5.

Lippitt's Dichotomy: Static vs. Future-Oriented Organizations.

	Characteristics	
Dimensions	*Static Organizations*	*Future-Oriented Organizations*
Structure	Rigid: permanent committees; reverence for constitution and bylaws, tradition Hierarchical: chain of command Role definitions: narrow Property: bound and restricted	Flexible: temporary task force; readiness to change constitution and bylaws, depart from tradition Linking: functional collaboration Role definitions: broad Property: mobile and regional
Atmosphere	Internally competitive Task-centered: reserved Cold, formal: aloof	Goal-oriented People-centered: caring Warm, informal: intimate
Management and Philosophy	Controlling: coercive power Cautious: low risk Errors: to be prevented Emphasis on personal selection Self-sufficient: closed system re: resources Emphasis on conserving resources Low tolerance for ambiguity	Releasing: supportive power Experimental: high risk Errors: to be learned from Emphasis on personnel development Interdependent: open system re: resources Emphasis on developing and using resources High tolerance for ambiguity
Decision-Making and Policy-Making	High participation at top, low at bottom Clear distinction between policy-making and execution Decision-making by legal mechanisms Decisions treated as final	Relevant participation by all those affected Collaborative policy-making and execution Decision-making by problem-solving Decisions treated as hypotheses to be tested
Communication	Restricted flow: constipated One-way: downward Feelings: repressed or hidden	Open flow: easy access Two-way: upward and downward Feelings: expressed

RESISTANCE TO CHANGE

Zander's discussion of the resistance to change identifies six conditions which he perceives as conducive to the development and perpetuation of resistance to change.[5]

Resistance can be expected if the nature of the change is not made clear to the people who are going to be influenced by the change. In childbirth education, the demands for change were often made by lay people or professionals, who did not fully understand what was being asked or how it would alter their own performance.

Different people will see different meaning in the proposed change. If the people involved in the change feel that the change is a threat to their job, their authority, or their territory, then they will resist even if they fully understand the change—for example, the nurse who sees the expectant father as another responsibility or the physician who dislikes "demands" from his patients.

Resistance can be expected when those influenced are caught in a jam between strong forces pushing them to make the change and strong forces deterring them against making the change.

Resistance may be expected to the degree that the persons influenced by the change have pressure put upon them to make the change and will decrease to the degree that these same persons are able to have some "say" in the nature or direction of the change. Institution of family-centered care by hospital directive has been proven to be a very ineffective way to bring about the behavior necessary to implement the concept.

Resistance may be expected if the change is made on personal grounds rather than impersonal requirements. Because childbirth education has been such an emotionally laden movement, some agency changes have been made because of personal preference of leadership in choosing people who are "believers." However, the change should be presented in terms of the relationship to the institution's goals and objectives rather than as an individual's bias.

5. Alvin Zander, "Resistance to Change—Its Analysis and Prevention" in Bartlett and Kayser *op. cit.* pp. 405–7.

Resistance may be expected if the change ignores the already established institutions in the group. The separation of nursery and postpartum nursing is frequently the basis for resistance to the implementation of family-centered care.

While these are only a few of the possible causes and examples of resistance to change, if they are handled with forethought and care, if their existence and importance in the planning of changes is acknowledged, then the probable success of the effort will be greatly increased. Change is very frightening to most people. How many new ideas have been turned aside with "You cannot do it that way because we have never done it before?" It is very safe to keep our own systems going. We know where we stand and what to expect. If the change planner can remove the element of the unknown as much as possible, then it is less likely to meet with resistance.

EXISTING ALTERNATIVES

Although the traditional hospitals have been slow in modifying care, there have developed other forms of maternity care that bode well for the future.

Homelike Birthing Room (Hospital-Based)

In those traditional hospitals that cannot offer full-service family-centered care to all patients, it is possible to set aside space for those parents who seek it. Developed by obstetrician Philip E. Sumner at Manchester Hospital, Manchester, Connecticut, the concept of a Lamaze Room is based on the clinical facilities used by Dr. Pierre Vellay in Paris (Fig. 12–6). The basic idea is to provide all the facilities needed for labor and delivery in as homelike an environment as possible. So, the Lamaze Room prototype provides a special labor bed in a room decorated with wall paper and pictures (Fig. 12–6D). The father-coach is provided with a comfortable chair and all the supplies necessary to carry out his role as labor coach. When delivery is imminent, the physician assists the mother into position, where she can deliver in relative comfort. The birth room offers all the elements parents seek; the opportunity to be together, working together with no last-minute dashing to be set in the cold, dehumanized delivery room. Mother, father, and baby can be together

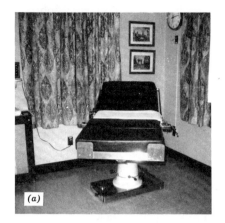 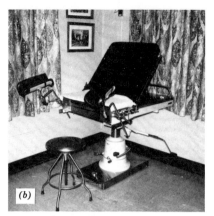

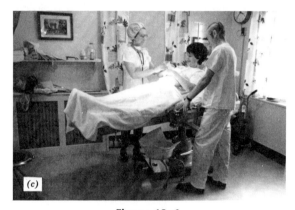

Figure 12-6.

(a) Labor/delivery bed imported from France. (Courtesy of Dr. P. Sumner.)
(b) Labor/delivery bed in delivery position. (Courtesy of Dr. P. Sumner.)
(c) The birthing room in use. (Courtesy of Dr. P. Sumner.)

immediately after birth for those all important minutes needed for bonding. Figure 12-7 shows examples of other birth rooms around the country.

The Childbearing Center

One alternative to traditional hospital maternity care is the childbearing center, set up as a demonstration project by Maternity Center Association in
(continued on page 207)

Figure 12-6. (d)

Program outline for the birthing room. (Reprinted by courtesy of Dr. Philip E. Sumner.)

THE BIRTHING ROOM—SAFE, JOYOUS CHILDBIRTH
Philip E. Sumner, MD   John P. Wheeler, MD   Samuel G. Smith, MD
Billie Carlson, RN, NP   Irma Meridy, RN, NP

In order for a prepared childbirth program to be fully effective a compatible and supportive environment is essential. Conventional maternity facilities and policies often disrupt, complicate, and prevent the psychoprophylactic (Lamaze) method from achieving maximum effectiveness which is then unfairly blamed on the method itself. The Homelike Labor-Delivery Room provides a compatible milieu for the psychoprophylactic method in which many different support systems—physical, physiological, psychological, emotional, aesthetic as well as medical—are synthesized and brought together to minimize the need for drugs and anesthetics and maximize the positive childbirth experience.

In 1969 Manchester Memorial Hospital established a fully equipped, homelike labor-delivery room in which prepared patients can labor, deliver, and remain together during the immediate postpartum period. The program has prospered to the benefit of all.

PROGRAM OUTLINE

I. *THE GOAL:*

    A. physically and emotionally healthy mother and baby
    B. positive delivery experience
    C. nonseparation of nuclear family

202

Figure 12–6. (*d*) (Continued)

II. *PREMISES:*

A. Childbirth is:
   1. fundamentally a normal physiological process
   2. a powerful emotional experience
   3. occasionally abnormal; therefore, hospital delivery is safer than home delivery

B. A *JOYOUS* MODEL IS PREFERABLE TO A *PATHOLOGICAL* MODEL
   1. Positive ambience decreases anxiety, facilitates labor
   2. Hospitals must provide both *safe* and *satisfying* childbirth
   3. A "high-risk" patient has even greater anxiety than a "low-risk" patient; therefore, a reassuring environment is even more essential.

C. The cornerstone of modern obstetric management is the patient's own mechanism of labor. Effective techniques can be learned so that most patients can become highly motivated to help themselves in labor (such as psychoprophylaxis or the "Lamaze" method).

D. Multiple noninvasive support systems are essential to minimize the need for "interference obstetrics" and maximize the childbirth experience.
   1. physically and emotionally prepared patient
   2. "prepared" husband or "significant other"
   3. private, attractive labor-delivery room
   4. a comfortable, functional labor-delivery bed
   5. constant one-to-one nursing support (monitrice)
   6. medical equipment "low profile," should not imply morbidity
   7. appropriate "backup" drugs and anesthetics
   8. in-place delivery
   9. sensitive period for optimum bonding
   10. celebration

E. A fully equipped, homelike labor-delivery room provides an appropriate milieu for the prepared childbirth patient in which the many different support systems are synthesized and brought together to reduce the risks, minimize intervention, and maximize the joy of childbirth.

Figure 12–6. (*d*) (Continued)

III. *FEATURES:*

A. *Prepared Childbirth (Lamaze) Classes*

1. Home classes provide warm, friendly, informal atmosphere
2. Held weekly last 6 weeks of pregnancy
3. Small size (4–6 couples) assures personalized attention
4. ASPO certified childbirth educators (Lamaze Method).[1]
5. Anatomy, physiology of pregnancy stressed but all aspects of family life and relationships covered
6. Relaxation, breathing, concentration, and proper pushing techniques taught
7. Husband (or "significant other") actively involved

B. *Homelike labor-delivery suite*

1. Attractive decor of colored wallpaper, drapes, pictures, mobile, bulletin board, large mirror, telephone, comfortable chair, reflects the positive emotions of childbirth
2. AM–FM radio provides musical background, record book (Lamaze log) records details of each delivery
3. Minimum patient distraction, disruption, and dislocation
4. Fully medically equipped; usual DR procedures and sterile techniques are followed (suction, oxygen, Kreizelman incubator, castle lamp on wall)
5. Located near regular DR in event of complication
6. Overhead lights are rheostated and may be dimmed after birth to encourage newborn–parent eye-to-eye contact
7. Heat panel;[2] prevents hypothermia while permitting extended skin-to-skin contact of mother and neonate

C. *Labor-delivery bed*[3]

1. Recognizes the physiological continuity of labor and delivery as two phases of a single event
2. Advantages of the labor-delivery bed
   a. To the patient:
      1. avoids the physical and emotional trauma of transfer
      2. permits continuity of concentration and control
      3. permits continuity of husband and monitrice support
      4. permits the nuclear family to remain in place for optimum "bonding"

1. ASPO: American Society for Psychoprophylaxis in Obstetrics (Lamaze Method) 1523 L St., Northwest, Washington, D.C. 20005
2. Air Shields Co., Hatboro, Pa. 19040
3. European LDB, Healthco Inc., 25 Stuart Street, Boston, MA 02116, manufactured by Pierre Mathieu & Cie, 16 Rue de Champ de l'Alouette, Paris 13, France

Figure 12–6. (*d*) (Continued)

b. To the physician:
  1. simplifies, expedites patient management
  2. continuous supervision of vital signs, fetal monitoring, IV solutions and medications and patient progress until delivery is completed
  3. eliminates unsterile precips on stretcher or in DR

c. To the nurse:
  1. eliminates the difficult decision of when to transfer
  2. eliminates the physical strain of transfer
  3. enables nurse to provide greater support and supervision
  4. economical use of nursing services

d. To the administration:
  1. maximum economy of space, staff and time for all
  2. eliminates reduplication of supplies, equipment
  3. favorable "progressive" hospital image

D. *Monitrice*[4]

1. Obstetric RN trained specifically in psychoprophylaxis (Lamaze method)
2. Provides continuous emotional and physical one-to-one support throughout labor and delivery (not necessarily available from staff nurses); she reinforces but does not usurp husband's role
3. Many are also childbirth educators (combines theory with practice)
4. 24 hour-a-day call roster
5. Coordinates at delivery with floor nurses
6. Not an employee of hospital, bills the patient directly
7. Provides a supplementary nursing service, thus helping to resolve the constant dilemma of "feast or famine" maternity staffing

E. *Medication and anesthesia—only if and when necessary*

1. systemic drugs discouraged—scopalomine never
2. anesthesia: regional, conduction, paracervical, pudendal, local all compatible
3. "modified" paracervical block is uniquely suitable: (2½ cc of 1% carbocaine injected through Iowa trumpet.[5] 1/8 inch submucosally in lateral vaginal fornixes at 3, 5, 7 and 9 o'clock—maximum 10 cc)

4. Manchester Monitrice Associates, 31 Bette Drive, Manchester, CT   06040
5. Iowa Trumpet: Distributed by Iowa Medical Supply Company, 9110 First Avenue, North, Fort Dodge, Iowa   50501

Figure 12–6. (*d*) (Continued)

a. may be given anytime during Stage I of labor
b. may be repeated hourly if necessary
c. given by obstetrician or nurse-midwife—*no anesthetist necessary*
d. dramatic, immediate effect
e. reduces, does not eliminate sensation—patient can still work with contractions
f. facilitates spontaneous delivery
g. minimal systemic effect—fetal bradycardia rare, no IV necessary

F. *In-place labor and delivery*

1. patient is ambulatory during labor, supine position avoided
2. vertex rotation attempted manually or by positional changes, forceps only when necessary
3. no dislocation of patient, personnel, or equipment
4. patient concentration, control not disturbed—birth position optional
5. patient may place legs in stirrups, lower half of bed pushed into upper half
6. wall light turned on, instrument table wheeled in
7. parents wash, wipe hands with facecloth
8. customary prep, drape except abdomen is exposed for skin-to-skin contact of mother and newborn
9. forceps, episiotomy, etc. only if necessary
10. neonate placed immediately on mother's abdomen, oral mucus aspirated if necessary, overhead light dimmed, heat panel turned on
11. mother may embrace and fondle baby immediately
12. Doctor changes gloves after cutting cord
13. placenta expelled spontaneously by patient, manual removal if necessary

G. *Sensitive period—first 60 minutes of life*[6]

1. neonate kept on mother's abdomen for maximum skin-to-skin contact
2. heat panel placed over baby and mother to prevent hypothermia (temp. at 20 + 40 min.)
3. breast contact encouraged
4. silver nitrate withheld until transfer

6. M. Klaus and J. Kennell, "Maternal-infant Bonding," (St. Louis: C. V. Mosby, 1976), pp. 50–66.

Figure 12–6. (d) (Continued)

5. "en-face" eye-to-eye bonding encouraged
6. father encouraged to hold neonate
7. appropriate celebration—pictures taken, phone calls made, champagne toast

H. *Family transferred together to recovery or postpartum room*

1. breast feeding, rooming-in, sibling visiting encouraged
2. postpartum classes for both father and mother
3. parents encouraged to assume responsibility, gain confidence
4. medical personnel are supportive, not autocratic
5. early ambulation, discharge encouraged

New York City and conducted by certified nurse-midwives. The primary goal is, "to provide safe, satisfying and economical care to couples who can anticipate a normal birth and wish to participate actively in the childbearing experience."

Parents are carefully screened for medical problems, after which they are thoroughly informed of the services and options open to them. Preparation in the form of individual and group classes is made available, and mothers and fathers—or any support person of the mother's choosing—are urged to participate (Fig. 12–8). Once in labor, the couple comes to the center. A physical examination is done to determine progress of labor (Fig. 12–9). Enemas and perineal preps are done only when indicated, not routinely. The mother is encouraged to walk around in early labor and enjoy the garden and family room where she can relax, read, play cards, or have light refreshment. Once labor is active, the couple retires to the labor/delivery room, where they will remain until discharge about 12 hours after delivery (Fig. 12–10). Parents are encouraged to inspect, touch, and cuddle their baby as soon as airway has been established and the infant wrapped for warmth (Fig. 12–11). A follow-up home visit is made about 24 hours after delivery and the mother and baby are seen at about one week and again at five to six weeks postpartum at the childbearing center.

The Family Hospital

The Family Hospital in Milwaukee, Wisconsin, is another alternative that could make family-centered care readily available in the future. It is a total hospital dedicated to the idea that families have the right to participate in the care of their loved ones during times of stress (Fig. 12–12). The unique

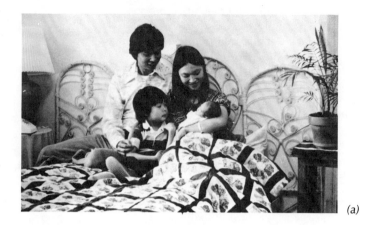

(a)

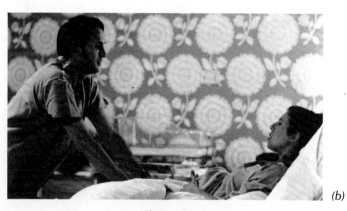

(b)

Figure 12–7.

(a) The Wong family admires its newest member at Mount Zion Alternative Birth Center in San Francisco. (Photo courtesy of Mount Zion Hospital and Medical Center.) (b) Mr. Harris assists his wife during labor in homelike birthing room at Phoenix's Memorial Hospital. (With permission of South Phoenix Ambulatory and Emergency Care Center.)

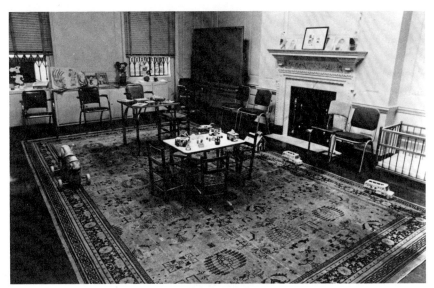

Figure 12–8.

This multipurpose room serves as a place where mothers can leave small children while they are being examined during the day and doubles as a classroom for parents at night. (Photo courtesy Maternity Center Association, New York, N.Y.)

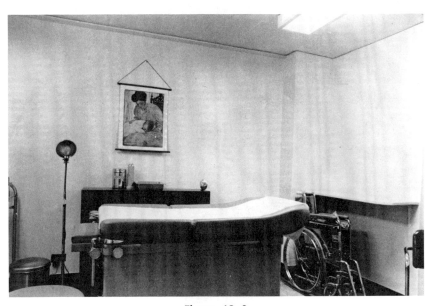

Figure 12–9.

Even in the examining room, there are attempts to add homelike touches. (Photo courtesy Maternity Center Association, New York, N.Y.)

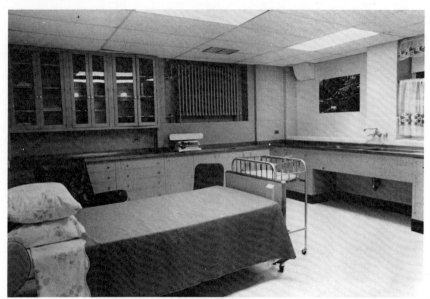

Figure 12–10.

A homelike labor/delivery room at the Childbearing Center. (Photo courtesy Maternity Center Association, New York, N.Y.)

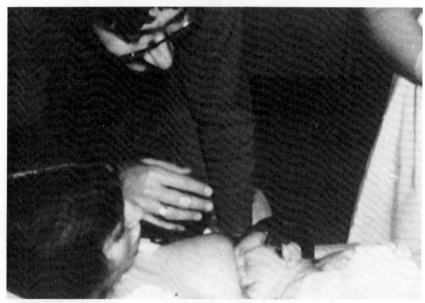

Figure 12–11.

As soon as the airway is established, parents are encouraged to hold and cuddle the infant. They may stay together until discharge which, if all goes well, is about 12 hours after delivery.

Figure 12–12.

A totally family-centered hospital.

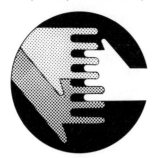

family hospital

FAMILY HOSPITAL
NURSING SERVICE DEPARTMENT

FAMILY-CENTERED CARE OVERVIEW

GOAL: Provision of family-centered care coordinated by the professional nurse in collaboration with the patient's physician and others.

RATIONALE: The professional nurse as care-planner and care-giver together with the patient and his family, is best qualified to identify patient needs and to develop a plan of action to meet those needs in the acute care setting. In this setting this care-giver is identified as the family care nurse, who has a direct responsibility to the patient and physician.

PREMISE: Family-centered care and professional nurse accountability naturally complement and enhance one another, therefore family care nursing is the best means by which our philosophy can be implemented.

PHILOSOPHY

PATIENT NEEDS: The patient, in order to maintain and preserve his dignity, self-respect, and integrity: a) needs to be an active participant-consultant in the planning and implementing of his care, b) needs information and education necessary to cope with the changes in his lifestyle resulting from hospitalization, c) needs the

Figure 12-12. (Continued)

mental and emotional support provided by those significant to him during a health crisis.

FAMILY NEEDS: The family, as intimately involved with the patient, needs to remain in close contact with, be educated and informed about, and participate, when possible, in the day-to-day care and progress of their family member.

STAFF NEEDS: The staff, as liaison between patient–family–physician— and allied health services, needs support, freedom, respect, and understanding as well as the recognition of his/her personal needs by the hospital organization. As staff needs are met the employee is then better prepared and motivated to meet the needs of patients and their families.

BASIC CONCEPTS OF
FAMILY-CENTERED NURSING

A. Assignment by responsible nurse of each patient to a specific family care nurse (FCN) who usually provides his care each day she is on duty until the patient's discharge or transfer.

B. Patient assessment by FCN, who plans his care using consultant nurses as necessary, and who communicates to an Associate FCN through written directives on kardex and other communication tools; thus 24-hour accountability.

C. Patient and family involvement in the care provided with identification of his goals relating to how the medical condition affects his lifestyle.

D. Care-giver to care-giver communication—both in the nursing staff's daily reporting methods and between disciplines.

E. Discharge planning—including patient and family teaching, family involvement, and appropriate referrals.

OBJECTIVES OF
FAMILY-CENTERED CARE

A. Family-Centered Care—to provide care in which the patient with his family is the central focus for planning care, implementing care, and evaluating care.

Figure 12-12. (Continued)

B. Accountability for Family-Centered Care—to assign staff and encourage the selection of patients and families by staff so that the most effective use is made of the individual's skills and knowledge through family-centered nursing, which is the assignment and accountability for the total nursing care of one patient and his family to a single nurse.

C. Continuity of Family-Centered Care—to provide for continuity of care by assigning one patient and his family to one FCN who coordinates the care by selecting Associate FCNs who follow through on the plan of care.

D. Comprehensive Family-Centered Care—to provide a holistic approach to family-centered care as opposed to a specialized approach to patient care.

E. Coordination of Family-Centered Care—to provide a congruous approach to patient and family in which the more global aspects of care are highlighted.

F. Staff Development—to encourage and facilitate the growth and knowledge of the nursing staff by providing relevant learning opportunities.

offering of this facility through its New Life Center is that in addition to providing for the mother and father, provisions are also made for other children and for grandparents. The total family is seen as a unit—interdependent and working together. Viewing the family this way, one can see that separation from the family is an added stress. Therefore, the New Life Center of the Family Hospital provides the many options from which the family can select depending on what their desires and needs are (Fig. 12-13).

OPTIONS FOR THE FUTURE

The future is upon us. The directions that are chosen today will become the history of tomorrow. Childbirth education has been in the forefront of the movement to humanize medical care. It has been there largely through the efforts of those parents who believed that it did make a difference in their confidence and ability to cope with the maturational crisis of becoming a parent. Professionals are latecomers to this movement. True, childbirth edu-

We present some of the options that you will probably want to decide on before, during and after childbirth. None of them are required by the hospital, and your decisions can be made (or changed) at any time you desire. This list is intended to serve as a guide to the choices available to you at the Center and for preparatory discussions with your family and physician.

during pregnancy, you may or may not choose to:
- tour the Center, visit with the staff and the new mothers
- attend the Center's information and instruction classes with your husband, friends or members of the family

during labor and delivery, you may or may not choose to:
- spend the early labor period walking around the lounge and watching TV
- have someone with you (husband, relative or friend) during labor and the baby's birth
- give birth in the traditional delivery room
- give birth in a private labor room
- be awake for your baby's delivery
- be asleep during your baby's delivery
- give birth in a semi-sitting position
- use stirrups for your legs during birth
- help determine your own need for medication for pain or tension
- view the birth process through a large overhead mirror
- hold your baby immediately after birth or during the first few hours
- photograph or tape record the birth
- have the baby and your husband spend the first few hours together with you
- breast feed your baby right after birth or during the first few hours

during your stay, you may or may not choose to:
- breast feed your baby
- bottle feed your baby
- have your baby with you for feedings only
- have your baby with you for long periods of time each day
- have your husband visit you at any time
- have our nursing staff bathe and care for your baby in your room rather than the nursery
- have our nursing staff help you, the father, or another member of the family learn the skills of bathing, feeding and caring for your baby
- bathe and care for your own baby with the assistance of our nursing staff
- have your shower at any time you prefer
- have the father or a visitor join you for meals
- have your other children visit you
- have your other children view the new baby
- if a boy, have the baby circumcised
- attend informal group discussions with other mothers and members of our nursing staff
- attend a series of films on baby care shown at the center

after returning home, you may or may not choose to:
- have a hospital staff member phone you to answer any questions you may have
- have a hospital staff member visit you at your home for additional instruction or to answer any questions you may have.
- attend discussion groups with other new mothers and members of our staff, see new films, hear guest speakers
- receive birth control information from our staff

Figure 12–13.

Choices at the New Life Center.

214

cation is an integral part of nursing, but nursing has been reactive, responding to the needs of parents rather than predicting the needs and preparing to meet them. The future is now. Unless we, the professionals, are willing to examine the options and take strong positions, someone else will do it for us. We cannot afford to wait for that to happen. Nursing is at a crossroads in time. Unless we are willing to choose and step confidently forward, we will be left behind.

BIBLIOGRAPHY

Abdellah F et al: *New Directions in Patient-Centered Nursing: Guidelines for Systems of Service, Education and Research.* New York, Macmillan Co, 1973.

Arms S: How Hospitals Complicate Childbirth, *MS,* May 1975.

Bean MA: Birth is a Family Affair, *American Journal of Nursing* **75**:10, Oct 1975.

Bennis WG et al: *The Planning of Change,* 2nd ed. New York, Holt, Rinehart and Winston, 1969.

Bertrard A: *Social Organization: A General Systems and Role Theory Perspective.* Philadelphia, F. A. Davis, 1972.

Brown MS: A Cross Cultural Look at Pregnancy, Labor and Delivery, *JOGN* **5**:5, Sep/Oct 1976.

Brozan N: Families Learn How to Provide Self-Help Care for Mothers-to-be, *New York Times,* Friday, March 17, 1978.

Cirz D: Nurses and the Future in Childbirth, *JOGN* **7**:1, Jan/Feb 1978.

Cornell EB: The Modern Nurse–Midwife, *Redbook,* July 1974.

Ferris C: The Alternative Birth Center at Mount Zion Hospital *Birth and the Family Journal,* Fall 1976.

Haggerty J: Woman's Body, Woman's Mind: Childbirth Made Difficult, *Ms,* January 1973.

Haire D: *The Cultural Warping of Childbirth.* Seattle, Wash, ICEA, 1972.

Hammerschmidt ES: The Editor Visits the New Life Center, *Baby Talk,* Nov 1975.

Home Oriented Maternity Experience, A Comprehensive Guide to *Home Birth,* Washington, DC, HOME, 1976.

Lang D: The Midwife Returns: Modern Style, *Parents Magazine,* Oct 1972.

Lewton M: Woman, Wife, Mother—What's Best for Newborns and Parents—Giving Birth in the Hospital or at Home, *Family Health,* Jan 1977.

Lubic RW: Comprehensive Maternity Care as An Ambulatory Service, *Journal of New York State Nurses Association,* vol 8, Nov/Dec 1977.

————, Developing Maternity Service Women Will Trust, *American Journal of Nursing*, **75**:10, Oct 1975.

McCleary EH: *New Miracles of Childbirth.* New York, David McKay, 1974.

Manchester Monitrice Associates: *The Birth of a Monitrice*, Manchester, Conn, MMA, 1978.

Muller JS: Return to the Joy of Home Delivery with Fathers in the Delivery Room, *Hospital Topics*, Jan 1966.

Parfitt RR: *The Birth Primer: Sourcebook of Traditional and Alternative Methods of Labor and Delivery*, 1977.

Roe A, Sherwood M: *Nursing in the Seventies.* New York, John Wiley & Sons, 1973.

Sasmor JL: The Nurse Midwife: A Partner in Progress, *American Baby,* Oct 1973.

Scaer R, Korte D: MOM Survey—Maternity Options for Mothers—What Do Women Want in Maternity Care? *Birth and the Family Journal*, **5**:1, Spring 1978.

Sousa M: *Childbirth at Home.* New York, Bantam Books, 1976.

Stewart D, Stewart, L. (eds): *Safe Alternative in Childbirth.* Chapel Hill, NC, NAPSAC, 1976.

Stimeling G: Will Common Delivery Practices Soon Become Malpractice?, *Journal of Legal Medicine*, May 1975.

Sumner PE et al: The Home-Like Labor Delivery Room, *Connecticut Medicine,* May 1976.

Sumner PE et al: Six Year Experience of Prepared Childbirth in a Home-Like Labor-Delivery Room, *Birth and the Family Journal*, Spring 1976.

Swanson LB, Ritchie AH, Childbirth Outside the Hospital . . . *American Journal of Maternal Child Nursing,* Nov/Dec 1976.

Timberlake, Bobbi: "The New Life Center," *American Journal of Nursing,* September 1975.

Walker H: *Nursing and Ritualistic Practice*, New York, The Macmillan Co, 1967.

APPENDIX A

The Pregnant Patient's Bill of Rights

American parents are becoming increasingly aware that well-intentioned health professionals do not always have scientific data to support common American obstetrical practices and that many of these practices are carried out primarily because they are part of medical and hospital tradition. In the last forty years many artificial practices have been introduced which have changed childbirth from a physiological event to a very complicated medical procedure in which all kinds of drugs are used and procedures carried out, sometimes unnecessarily, and many of them potentially damaging for the baby and even for the mother. A growing body of research makes it alarmingly clear that every aspect of traditional American hospital care during labor and delivery must now be questioned as to its possible effect on the future well-being of both the obstetric patient and her unborn child.

One in every 35 children born in the United States today will eventually be diagnosed as retarded; in 75% of these cases there is no familial or genetic predisposing factor. One in every 10 to 17 children has been found to have some form of brain dysfunction or learning disability requiring special treatment. Such statistics are not confined to the lower socioeconomic group but cut across all segments of American society.

New concerns are being raised by childbearing women because no one knows what degree of oxygen depletion, head compression, or traction by forceps the unborn or newborn infant can tolerate before that child sustains

Prepared by Doris Haire, Chair., ICEA Committee on Health Law and Regulation permanent brain damage or dysfunction. The recent findings regarding the cancer-related drug diethylstilbestrol have alerted the public to the fact that neither the approval of a drug by the U.S. Food and Drug Administration nor the fact that a drug is prescribed by a physician serves as a guarantee that a drug or medication is safe for the mother or her unborn child. In fact, the American Academy of Pediatrics' Committee on Drugs has recently stated that there is no drug, whether prescription or over-the-counter remedy, which has been proven safe for the unborn child.

The pregnant patient has the right to participate in decisions involving her well-being and that of her unborn child, unless there is a clearcut medical emergency that prevents her participation. In addition to the rights set forth in the American Hospital Association's "Patient's Bill of Rights," (which has also been adopted by the New York City Department of Health) the pregnant patient, because she represents TWO patients rather than one, should be recognized as having the additional rights listed below.

1. *The pregnant patient has the right*, prior to the administration of any drug or procedure, to be informed by the health professional caring for her of any potential direct or indirect effects, risks, or hazards to herself or her unborn or newborn infant which may result from the use of a drug or procedure prescribed for or administered to her during pregnancy, labor, birth, or lactation.

2. *The pregnant patient has the right*, prior to the proposed therapy, to be informed, not only of the benefits, risks, and hazards of the proposed therapy but also of known alternative therapy, such as available childbirth education classes which could help to prepare the pregnant patient physically and mentally to cope with the discomfort or stress of pregnancy and the experience of childbirth, thereby reducing or eliminating her need for drugs and obstetric intervention. She should be offered such information early in her pregnancy in order that she may make a reasoned decision.

3. *The pregnant patient has the right*, prior to the administration of any drug, to be informed by the health professional who is prescribing or administering the drug to her that any drug which she receives during pregnancy, labor, and birth, no matter how or when the drug is taken or administered, may adversely affect her unborn baby, directly or indirectly, and that there is no drug or chemical which has been proven safe for the unborn child.

4. *The pregnant patient has the right* if Cesarean birth is anticipated, to be informed prior to the administration of any drug, and preferably prior to

her hospitalization, that minimizing her and, in turn, her baby's intake of nonessential preoperative medicine will benefit her baby.

5. *The pregnant patient has the right*, prior to the administration of a drug or procedure, to be informed of the areas of uncertainty if there is NO properly controlled follow-up research which has established the safety of the drug or procedure with regard to its direct and/or indirect effects on the physiological, mental, and neurological development of the child exposed, via the mother, to the drug or procedure during pregnancy, labor, birth, or lactation. This would apply to virtually all drugs and the vast majority of obstetric procedures.

6. *The pregnant patient has the right*, prior to the administration of any drug, to be informed of the brand name and generic name of the drug in order that she may advise the health professional of any past adverse reaction to the drug.

7. *The pregnant patient has the right* to determine for herself, without pressure from her attendant, whether she will accept the risks inherent in the proposed therapy or refuse a drug or procedure.

8. *The pregnant patient has the right* to know the name and qualifications of the individual administering a medication or procedure to her during labor or birth.

9. *The pregnant patient has the right* to be informed, prior to the administration of any procedure, whether that procedure is being administered to her for her or her baby's benefit (medically indicated) or as an elective procedure (for convenience, teaching purposes, or research).

10. *The pregnant patient has the right* to be accompanied during the stress of labor and birth by someone she cares for, and to whom she looks for emotional comfort and encouragement.

11. *The pregnant patient has the right* after appropriate medical consultation to choose a position for labor and for birth which is least stressful to her baby and to herself.

12. *The obstetric patient has the right* to have her baby cared for at her bedside if her baby is normal, and to feed her baby according to her baby's needs rather than according to the hospital regimen.

13. *The obstetric patient has the right* to be informed in writing of the name of the person who actually delivered her baby and the professional qualifications of that person. This information should also be on the birth certificate.

14. *The obstetric patient has the right* to be informed if there is any known or indicated aspect of her or her baby's care or condition which may cause her or her baby later difficulty or problems.

15. *The obstetric patient has the right* to have her baby's hospital medical records complete, accurate and legible and to have their records, including Nurses' Notes, retained by the hospital until the child reaches at least the age of majority, or, alternatively, to have the records offered to her before they are destroyed.

16. *The obstetric patient*, both during and after her hospital stay, has the right to have access to her complete hospital medical records, including Nurses' Notes, and to receive a copy upon payment of a reasonable fee and without incurring the expense of retaining an attorney.

It is the obstetric patient and her baby, not the health professional, who must sustain any trauma or injury resulting from the use of a drug or obstetric procedure. The observation of the rights listed above will not only permit the obstetric patient to participate in the decisions involving her and her baby's health care, but will help to protect the health professional and the hospital against litigation arising from resentment or misunderstanding on the part of the mother.

The Pregnant Patient's Responsibilities

In addition to understanding her rights the pregnant patient should also understand that she too has certain responsibilities. The pregnant patient's responsibilities include the following:

1. The pregnant patient is responsible for learning about the physical and psychological process of labor, birth, and postpartum recovery. The better informed expectant parents are, the better they will be able to participate in decisions concerning the planning of their care.
2. The pregnant patient is responsible for learning what comprises good prenatal and intranatal care and for making an effort to obtain the best care possible.
3. Expectant parents are responsible for knowing about those hospital policies and regulations which will affect their birth and postpartum experience.
4. The pregnant patient is responsible for arranging for a companion or support person (husband, mother, sister, friend, etc.) who will share in her plans for birth and who will accompany her during her labor and birth experience.
5. The pregnant patient is responsible for making her preferences known clearly to the health professionals involved in her case in a courteous and cooperative manner and for making mutually agreed-upon arrangements regarding maternity care alternatives with her physician and hospital in advance of labor.
6. Expectant parents are responsible for listening to their chosen physician

Prepared by Members of ICEA. Published by International Childbirth Education Association, Inc. For a complimentary copy send a stamped, self-addressed envelope to Box 1900, New York, NY 10001. Bulk orders available from ICEA Publication/Distribution Center, P. O. Box 9316, Midtown Plaza, Rochester, NY 14604.

or midwife with an open mind, just as they expect him or her to listen openly to them.

7. Once they have agreed to a course of health care, expectant parents are responsible, to the best of their ability, for seeing that the program is carried out in consultation with others with whom they have made the agreement.

8. The pregnant patient is responsible for obtaining information in advance regarding the approximate cost of her obstetric and hospital care.

9. The pregnant patient who intends to change her physician or hospital is responsible for notifying all concerned, well in advance of the birth if possible, and for informing both of her reasons for changing.

10. In all their interactions with medical and nursing personnel, the expectant parents should behave towards those caring for them with the same respect and consideration they themselves would like.

11. During the mother's hospital stay the mother is responsible for learning about her and her baby's continuing care after discharge from the hospital.

12. After birth, the parents should put into writing constructive comments and feelings of satisfaction and/or dissatisfaction with the care (nursing, medical and personal) they received. Good service to families in the future will be facilitated by those parents who take the time and responsibility to write letters expressing their feelings about the maternity care they received.

All the previous statements assume a normal birth and postpartum experience. Expectant parents should realize that, if complications develop in their cases, there will be an increased need to trust the expertise of the physician and hospital staff they have chosen. However, if problems occur, the childbearing woman still retains her responsibility for making informed decisions about her care or treatment and that of her baby. If she is incapable of assuming that responsibility because of her physical condition, her previously authorized companion or support person should assume responsibility for making informed decisions on her behalf.

APPENDIX B

Interprofessional Task Force on Health Care of Women and Children: Policies on Family-Centered Childbirth

1. All hospitals should offer birth preparation classes for both mothers and fathers, including instruction on breast feeding and the role men can play in delivery.
2. Fathers should be permitted to accompany women giving birth during the entire process, including being present in the delivery room and helping with the birth itself. There should be no restriction of this privilege if the two parents are not married.
3. Hospitals would offer parents the option of using a homelike "birthing room" rather than a standard delivery room. The birthing room would contain informal furnishings and bear little resemblance to a surgical facility, as delivery rooms do.
4. There would be an end to restrictions—some spelled out by state law or health department regulation—on young children visiting their mothers and newborn siblings in the hospital.
5. Hospitals would develop programs to accelerate the release of mothers after birth so the newborn and its mother could quickly move back into the more psychologically secure atmosphere of the home. Hospitals would probably have to develop programs in which health professionals visited mothers and new babies in the home.

Similar papers have been developed by the American Nurses Association, the American College of Nurse Midwives, the American College of Obstetricians and Gynecologists and the American Academy of Pediatrics.

Reported by Myryame Montrose, "New Options in Childbirth: Part I Family-Centered Care" *American Baby Magazine*, May 1978, p. 50.

223

APPENDIX C

The following are samples of childbirth education teaching outlines. Each represents a different style of planning and teaching; each is aimed at a different target population of expectant parents.

Expectant and New Mothers' Course Teaching Outline (for adolescent mothers)
> Part One: Prenatal Classes and Handouts
> Part Two: Parenting Classes and Handouts

Prepared Childbirth Teaching Outline (Couples Classes)
> Part One: St. Anthony's Hospital, Inc. Prepared Childbirth Class Outline
> Part Two: Course Outline

Expectant and New Mothers' Course Teaching Outline

INSTRUCTORS

JONNA JUNG, RN, BS
Childbirth Educator
Sarasota County Health Dept.

JANET GAUVAIN, RN, BS
Childbirth Educator
Sarasota County Health Dept.

PART ONE
PRENATAL CLASSES AND HANDOUTS

1. TARGET POPULATION

This course is designed for low-income expectant mothers who have no resources available for private prenatal care. By having the class meetings in the neighborhood, it is hoped to facilitate greater attendance by reducing the need for transportation.

2. COURSE DESCRIPTION

The Expectant Mothers' Course is provided for all expectant mothers attending the Sarasota County Health Department Obstetrical Clinic. A series of

227

twelve classes will be provided. Oral presentations, follow-up discussions, films, literature, and neuromuscular control exercises will be utilized for instructing those expectent mothers from one to five months of pregnancy. Breathing techniques will be added during the sixth to ninth months of gestation. After the initial series of six to eight classes, the expectant mothers from the sixth to ninth month of pregnancy will be shown how to develop skills in neuromuscular control and breathing techniques.

3.   COURSE OUTLINES

Class locations may vary with different series of classes, depending on needs of expectant mothers. Current locations and times include:

3. 1.

Location	Day	Time
Payne Chapel	Wednesday	10:30 AM–12:30 PM
Booker School	Friday	3–5 PM
S. C. H. D.	Thursday	1–3 PM
Colson Avenue Church	Monday	2:30–4:30 PM

4.   PRIMARY LEARNING NEEDS:

4. 1. Immediate application of learned concepts to the client's real-life situation in this maturational crisis (Hall, 1974).

4. 2. Improved communication skills (AJN. 9–1975, p. 1502).

4. 3. Allow dependency as a step in maturation (AJN. 9–1975, p. 1502).

4. 4. Productive interpersonal relations (Spradley, 1975, p. 179).

4. 5. More concrete, less abstract approach (Knowles, 1970).

4. 6. Improved self-esteem (Hall, 1974, pp. 51–63 and Murray and Zentner, 1975, pp. 170–74).

4. 7. Progress in self-actualization potential (Murray and Zentner, 1975, p. 179).

5. COURSE OBJECTIVES:

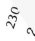

This prenatal course is designed to meet the needs of low-inc..
mothers in the following ways:

5. 1. Provide an atmosphere conducive to establishing a trusting relationship which will generate feelings of self-worth and foster expressions
of feelings.

5. 2. Provide basic knowledge of female anatomy and physiology related
to pregnancy, labor, and delivery.

5. 3. Provide information on nutrition, its importance during pregnancy
and application of learned facts related to the individual's lifestyle.

5. 4. Exploring minor complications of pregnancy and myths related to
their occurrence and treatment.

5. 5. Discussion of "risks" of pregnancy, leading into a discussion of more
serious complications of pregnancy.

5. 6. Present basic neuromuscular control exercises and breathing techniques in an effort to facilitate greater relaxation and conservation of
energy during the labor and delivery processes.

5. 7. Provide information on the processes of labor and delivery. Relate
specific exercises and breathing techniques to these processes.

5. 8. Provide information on and compare the advantages/disadvantages
of breast and bottle feeding.

5. 9. Explore various methods and reasons for family planning.

5. 10. Generate awareness for making family adjustments when the new
baby arrives home.

5. 11. Facilitate a discussion of physical, social, and emotional need of
newborns and their mothers.

Conception

LEARNER OBJECTIVES:

The client will:

1. Identify at least four female sex organs involved in conception and/or
reproduction.

. Describe at least one function for each of these organs.

3. Define conception and the relationship to ovulation.

4. State the basis for lack of menstruation, as a normal process during pregnancy with temporary cessation of subsequent fertilization for the duration of pregnancy.

5. Identify the structures involved with the developing fetus on an unlabeled illustration.

6. Examine the relationship of the placenta to the uterus and fetus.

7. Examine illustrations of initial conception in comparison with progressing fetal development.

8. Also examine the abilities of the fetus in regard to developmental activities.

9. Perform prenatal physical exercises (Kaegal, Taylor sitting, isometric adductor stretching, squatting, pelvic rock, modified leg lifts and relaxation).

TEACHING STRATEGIES:

The instructors will:

1. Present and discuss anatomical illustrations (ovaries, fallopian tubes, uterus, cervix, vagina) of organs involved in conception through the use of:

2. "Understanding" (Ortho Pharmaceutical Corp), "Conception" (Parke-Davis), and "Female Reproductive Organs" (Tampax, Inc.)

3. Describe the process of ovulation, conception, and normal termination of menses during pregnancy through the use of the film "Human Growth and Development #3" or alternate film and discussion.

4. Discuss the structures involved in the formation of the developing fetus and their functions (placenta, umbilical cord, amniotic sac, uterus, and cervix).

5. Stimulate a discussion of anovulation during pregnancy.

6. Present varying stages of fetal growth and development by using the Birth Atlas, Chart of Baby's Prental Growth and film **"When Life Begins."**

7. Demonstrate exercises listed in learner objective number 9.

EVALUATION

1. Feedback of clients through discussion by end of class time.
2. Clients will verbalize four female reproductive organs and at least one function of each by end of class time.
3. Clients will complete an unlabeled diagram of these reproduction organs (i.e., ovary, fallopian tubes, uterus, cervix and vagina) during class time.
4. Monitoring and appraisal of muscle tone during performance of exercises during class time.

SOURCES USED:

Film: "When Life Begins."
"Baby's Prenatal Growth Chart" Pampers.
"Female Reproductive Organs" Tampax Corp.
"How the Pill Works" Illustrations.
Nilsson: *A Child is Born.* New York, Delacorte Press, 1977.
Sasmor J: *What Every Husband Should Know About Having a Baby.* Chicago, Nelson-Hall, 1972.

Nutrition

LEARNER OBJECTIVES:

1. The clients will demonstrate knowledge of the four basic food groups and food sources they are found in.
2. The clients will demonstrate knowledge of the relationship of good nutrition (as evidenced by the four basic food groups) to their pregnancy by answering the following questions:

2. 1.   What are the four basic food groups?

2. 2.   What is a "serving"?

2. 3.   "Eating for two" is often expressed. What do we mean by that?

2. 3. 1. Completion of the weight gain grid.

3. The clients will demonstrate awareness of the nutritional needs of adolescents compounded by pregnancy as evidenced by discussion of rapid growth during adolescence plus the growth of the fetus.

4. The client will verbalize the need for specific vitamins and minerals during pregnancy.

TEACHING STRATEGIES:

1. The instructors will identify the clients' present knowledge of the four basic food groups through informal discussion.

2. The instructors will present information on the four basic food groups, clarifying with examples of each. Illustration of food charts will be used to reinforce presentation.

3. A library of literature containing at least eight sources of nutrition information will be available to clients to take home for a one-week period.

4. The instructors will emphasize the importance of specific vitamins and minerals necessary for mother and fetus, ie folic acid, iron, and calcium and sources for each.

5. The instructors will initiate a discussion of quantity vs. quality, and special importance of nutrition to the adolescent expectant mother.

6. The instructors will utilize one of the two films: "Great Expectations" or "Eating for Two" or filmstrip "Inside my Mom" to reinforce discussions.

7. The instructors will utilize informal group discussion after the presentation and films to assess learning.

8. The instructors will avoid giving advice and making value judgments.

9. The instructors will utilize personal nutritional data sheets for students to complete.

10. After two weeks, review of #9 will be done in class, objectively using guidelines from #2 to determine improvements.

11. The instructors will request each client to complete a personal weight grid comparing her pattern of weight gain to a standard pattern.

12. The instructors will utilize opportunities in subsequent classes to demonstrate the relatedness of nutrition to other aspects of pregnancy (eg, complications) and maintain the importance of continuity throughout pregnancy (and even lifetime).

METHOD OF EVALUATION:

1. Feedback through discussions.
2. Completion and review of nutritional data sheets.
3. Monitoring of weight grid pattern.

Female Pelvic Anatomy

LEARNER OBJECTIVE:

1. The client will verbalize basic knowledge of female pelvic anatomy and physiology related to pregnancy by termination of the course.
2. The client will describe the stress on the organs with the increased size of the uterus by termination of the course.
3. The client will verbalize her feelings regarding vaginal examination by the end of this class session.
4. The client will describe the rationale for minor complications experienced during pregnancy by end of class session (ie frequency, constipation, indigestion, flatus, backache, leg aches/cramps and restlessness).

TEACHING STRATEGIES

The instructor will:
1. Assess clients' present knowledge of female pelvic anatomy as evidenced by their ability to identify at least two landmarks on the female pelvic model.

2. Utilize informal group discussion in presenting female pelvic anatomical landmarks.
3. Utilize visual aids (pelvic model, film, and illustrations) for reinforcement of pelvic anatomy.
4. Promote an atmosphere conducive to free expression and asking questions.
5. Describe the changing anatomy that occurs with the progression of pregnancy that produces stress on adjacent pelvic organs.
6. Identify and promote a discussion of the resulting physical symptoms from the enlarging uterus.
7. Relate #6 to clients' own discomforts and introduce measures possible to alleviate symptoms.
8. Generate a discussion of changing breast structure.

EVALUATION

1. Verbal feedback of clients after presentation of information has been completed.
2. Demonstration of clients' ability to identify pelvic organs on pelvic model or illustrations.
3. Demonstrate competence in performing prenatal exercises and relaxation techniques.

SOURCES USED:

Bing E: *Moving Thru Pregnancy*. New York, Bobbs-Merrill, 1975.
Jensen M: *Maternity Care*. St. Louis, C. V. Mosby Co, 1977.
"Birth Atlas." New York, Maternity Center.
"Pregnancy—in Anatomical Illustrations." Carnation Company, 1965.
"Prenatal Care." U. S. D. H. E. W. 1973.
"What to do About Minor Discomforts of Pregnancy?" Ross Laboratories, 1975.
Film: "The Waiting Months" (Med Fact)

Early Pregnancy

LEARNER OBJECTIVES:

The client will:

1. progress toward meeting new developmental tasks.
2. develop awareness and progress with ability to accept added responsibilities.
3. recognize and determine changes necessary in life/family situations due to pregnancy.
4. recognize available community agencies that can help with specific problems.

TEACHING STRATEGIES:

The instructors will:

1. provide an atmosphere that is conducive for clients to explore and express feelings freely.
2. stimulate and guide clients toward independent thinking and decision-making.
3. identify community agencies and discuss their possible methods of support for these clients:
   eg
   - Social and Economic Services
   - Food Stamps
   - WIC
   - County Welfare
   - S. O. L. V. E.
   - Salvation Army
   - Family Counseling Association
4. present film: "Lucy."

5. explore reaction of client, family, infants' father, and peers to the pregnancy.
6. invite resource personnel that have expertise in psychosocial guidance, eg Marilyn Stover and/or Ms. McKenna.

EVALUATION:

1. Feedback through discussion.
2. Evidence of gradual progression of growth from dependency toward independent decision-making by termination of course.
3. Clients will list at least two changes they have made or will make related to their pregnancy.

Danger Signs to Watch For

IMPORTANCE

There are certain conditions that are of importance to the doctor. Should any of these occur, try to phone your doctor immediately. They may not indicate any serious condition, but only your doctor can determine this.

SIGNS

1. Vaginal bleeding or spotting
2. Swelling or puffing of the face, hands, or ankles
3. Persistent vomiting
4. Persistent daily headaches
5. Blurring of vision or spots before your eyes
6. Uncontrollable leakage of water from the vagina

7. Any sharp pain that persists with or without bleeding
8. Chills and fever
9. Marked increase or decrease in the amount of urine passed or burning on urination
10. Sudden weight gain

Labor and Delivery

LEARNER OBJECTIVES:

The client will:

1. Identify current knowledge and attitudes about labor and the birth process during this class session.
2. Recognize an alternative childbirth method (ie psychoprophylactic) by the end of this childbirth course.
3. State the difference between true and false labor contractions during this class session.
4. Identify three symptoms signaling the onset of true labor by termination of this course.
5. Verbalize her learned responses to the onset of true labor by termination of this course.
6. Discuss the initial activities that begin upon her arrival in the labor room during this class session.
7. Identify the three stages of labor and discuss characteristics of each stage by termination of the course.
8. Describe the processes of dilatation and effacement during this class session.
9. Verbalize the benefits of prenatal muscle exercises to the effectiveness of muscle tone during labor and delivery by end of this course.
10. Verbalize the benefits of other psychoprophylactic measures useful during labor and delivery by the end of this course.
11. Discuss her appropriate responses to each phase of labor by end of this course.
12. Perform exercises of concentration, relaxation, and breathing techniques specific to phases of labor and delivery at each class session.

13. Explore various types of analgesia and anesthetics commonly used in the local hospital during labor and delivery by the end of this class session.

TEACHING STRATEGIES:

The instructor will:

1. Initiate a discussion of commonly held beliefs and attitudes regarding labor and delivery.
2. Teach the psychoprophylactic methods of childbirth education.
3. Explain differences between true and false labor.
4. Describe those symptoms signaling the onset of true labor, leading into a discussion of when to go to the hospital.
5. Introduce psychoprophylactic measures and proper utilization of these measures at appropriate stages of labor.
6. Stimulate a discussion of those initial activities begun after admission to the labor room, ie shave and prep, enema, and pelvic exam.
7. Explain the stages and processes involved in labor and delivery.
8. Instruct in appropriate relaxation, concentration, and breathing techniques specific to stages of labor.
9. Discuss the benefits for psychoprophylactic techniques used in this prepared childbirth course.
10. Request presentation by either an obstetrician or anesthesiologist on types of analgesia and anesthesia commonly used during labor and delivery at either this class or next class session.

EVALUATION:

1. Feedback of clients through discussion by end of class session.
2. Clients will verbalize the three signs of true labor and state her response.
3. Clients will describe the processes of effacement, dilatation, and three stages of labor.

4. Monitoring and appraisal of neuromuscular exercises and breathing techniques.

SOURCES USED:

Literature packet on psychoprophylactic technique.
Bing E: *Moving Through Pregnancy.* New York, Bobbs-Merrill, 1975.
Dick-Read G MD: *Childbirth Without Fear.* New York, Harper & Row, 1970.
Jensen et al: *Maternity Care.* St. Louis, C. V. Mosby Co, 1977.
Film: Lynn and Smitty.

Process of Labor and Delivery

FIRST STAGE OF LABOR

A. Dilatation Stage
1. This period begins with the onset of true labor contractions and ends with complete dilatation of the cervix (10 cm).
B. Duration
1. Anywhere from 2–16 or more hours.
C. Characteristics
1. Uterine contractions which may follow a regular pattern and may be accompanied by:
a. rupture of the bag of waters
b. show (blood-tinged mucoid vaginal discharge)
D. What the Mother May Do
First baby: Lie down—time contractions.
1. Call the doctor when one or more symptoms of labor are present, or when you are in doubt, or when there is any change in the situation since you last reported to him.
2. Go to the hospital as the doctor advises or immediately if onset of labor is rapid.

3. Do not start relaxation and breathing until your labor is well established or you begin to mind your contractions.
4. If remaining at home for a period of time, carry on with normal activities if possible, or keep diverted with other activities of interest.
5. When the doctor or nurse does a rectal examination relax the pelvic floor and do deep chest breathing.

E. How the Mother May Feel
1. You may feel excited as you can now expect that long-awaited baby.
2. As your labor progresses and if you have discomfort you may feel more apprehension and growing seriousness about this labor. This has been noted when mothers are about 4–5 cm or in other words when you are halfway dilated. Remember to continue your confidence in the people caring for you and follow the instructions given to you in class and by hospital personnel.

TRANSITIONAL STAGE

A. Definition
1. Part of the first stage of labor when the cervix is nearing complete dilatation.
B. Duration
1. Usually last through *10–20 contractions*
C. Characteristics
1. The uterine contractions may become stronger, longer, and MAY BE accompanied by some of the following signs:
   a. Cramps of shaking of the legs
   b. Generalized discomfort or apprehension
   c. Hiccoughing or belching
   d. Nausea or possibly vomiting
   e. Pulling or stretching sensation deep in the pelvis
   f. Rupture of the bag of waters if it has not done so previously
   g. Severe low backache
   h. Amnesia or desire to sleep
   i. Breathing becomes more rapid and noisy

D. How the Mother May Feel
   1. Increased apprehension and physical discomfort may be noted during this period due to the increase of the contractions.
   2. Many times you may feel that you don't want to be left alone and yet you may be irritated at the people around you or the procedures being done. The people caring for you recognize this and will help you as much as possible but try to relax and follow their instructions. Do not become discouraged, keeping in mind that this stage lasts only a short time.

SECOND STAGE OF LABOR

A. Expulsive Stage
   1. This period begins with the complete dilation of the cervix and ends with the birth of the baby.
B. Duration
   1. Anywhere from a few minutes to several hours.
C. Characteristics
   1. Contractions which may be two to three minutes apart becoming increasing expulsive in nature.
   2. There may be increased show.
   3. Desire to bear down.
D. What the Mother May Do
   1. Notify the nurse of desire to bear down.
   2. *Do not push unless directed to do so by the doctor or nurse.*
   3. Pushing is done at the height of the contraction and maintained throughout the duration of the contraction.
   4. Relax in between contractions.
   5. Pant when asked to do so or when asked not to push.
   6. Medications may be taken at this time to relieve discomfort if necessary.
E. How The Mother May Feel
   1. Relief of discomfort is usually obtained when pushing.
   2. You may find yourself very tired after each push and so it is essential to do general body relaxation to gain strength for the next contraction.

3. Many times it is hard to follow directions because of natural amnesia that accompanies this period.
4. A stretching or burning sensation may be felt due to the extreme vaginal stretching when the baby's head is being born but this will disappear rapidly.

THIRD STAGE

A. Placental Stage
   1. This stage begins with the birth of the baby and ends with the expulsion of the placenta and membranes.
B. Duration
   1. Anywhere from one to twenty minutes.
C. Characteristics
   1. Contractions temporarily cease upon the birth of the baby.
   2. When they resume, they usually are painless and are needed for the expulsion of the placenta.
D. What the Mother May Do
   1. Relax as much as possible.
   2. She may be asked to help push the placenta out.
E. How the Mother May Feel
   1. Tired but feeling a great sense of achievement.
   2. Usually is eager to hear and see her baby.
   3. Hungry and thirsty due to the energy used during the preceding stages.

Prepared Childbirth: Definition and Benefits

"Prepared Childbirth" means the training of both the mind and the body for more active participation in childbirth. The practice of good body mechanics, the use of relaxation and breathing techniques, plus an understanding of the process of birth help to eliminate fear and tension in labor and thus reduce pain. When severe pain is absent, and interested moral support and encouragement are present, mothers go through labor with less need for drugs or anesthetic.

THE BENEFITS

1. Greater comfort during pregnancy because of improved posture and more relaxed physical and mental attitude.
2. More comfortable, and on the average shorter labor, than an untrained labor would be.
3. A sense of supreme accomplishment in having actively shared and participated in the miracle of creating and producing a new life.
4. More rapid physical recovery from the effort of labor than a mother would otherwise have, and also a more rapid recovery generally. Breast feeding helps the uterus to return more rapidly to normal.

Psychoprophylactic Principles

1. It is not "natural childbirth," natural referring to the instinctive and without ability to control or alter behavior. For instance, a dog at term has her instincts aroused, so she looks for a place for her delivery and even prepares it. When labor begins, the dog goes to her nest, delivers young, bites the cord, cleans the young, puts them to the breast, and eats the placenta. THIS IS NATURAL.
2. Margaret Mead says that attitudes toward and behavior in childbirth are socially determined.
3. Within limits, each woman will experience childbirth in a roughly predictable fashion, depending upon the social grouping from which she comes and in which she has learned how one behaves under given circumstances.
4. The corollary is that human behavior patterns in childbirth can be unlearned as well, and new patterns, more or less efficient than the old, can be substituted.
5. The basis for the effect of psychoprophylaxis is: The brain can accept, integrate, interpret, and emanate only ONE set of signals at a time. If the

strongest set of signals arriving at the brain comes from the uterus and is interpreted as pain, the forthcoming behavioral response is apt to be: writhing, moaning, groaning, and perhaps weeping.

6. But if at the instant of the uterine contraction a series of actions is initiated that requires for its successful execution stronger signals than those the uterus sends, then the uterine signals assume second place and the conscious perception of the uterine contractions diminish markedly.

7. The exercises provide the strong set of stimuli necessary to take precedence over the signals from the uterine contractions.

Exercises

Relaxation and Concentration:

Lie in a comfortable position. Use pillows under head, back, or legs to promote comfort. Use your mind to think about various parts of your body, in order to relax.

Start with the feet and make them relax. Next think about your legs and make them relax. Continue up to the abdomen, then the chest, arms, neck and face making each part relax as you go. When you have relaxed each part, *feel* the relaxation in the body. If there is any part not relaxed, go back to that part and relax those muscles. Enjoy the feeling!

Practice this once or twice daily. This is especially good to practice before going to sleep at night.

PRINCIPLES

1. These exercises are designed to teach control of specific muscle groups—to condition the ability to use specific muscle groups to the exclusion of all others.

2. These exercises will not be used in labor—they are important preparations for techniques that will be used.

3. Repeat this series at least daily. Contractions and relaxations should be as complete as possible.

BODY BUILDING EXERCISES

PRINCIPLES

1. Not used as such during labor.
2. Designed to help stretch muscle groups that will be used extensively in labor and also help stretch the muscles of the outlet of the birth canal.
3. While performing, inhale through nose and exhale through mouth.
4. Perform *at least* once a day.

I.   TAILOR SIT

Position: Seated upright on the floor.

Method:

a. While seated upright on the floor, place soles of the feet together with the feet as close to the body as possible. Press your knees gently against the palms of your hand while applying upward pressure with your palms. Repeat about ten times. This exercise will increase the stretch of your ligaments.

II.   PELVIC ROCKING ON THE BACK

Position:

• Lie on back with knees bent. Hold feet and knees together.
• Place hands on front of hip bones.

Method:

a. Contract the muscles of the buttocks and at the same time pull the lower abdominal muscles inward and upward; hold; feel the small of the back come closer to the floor.

b. Relax the muscles of the buttocks and the lower abdominal muscles, at the same time arching the lower back, making a tunnel under it. This rocks the pelvis forward—front down and back up.

Suggestions and Values:

• It is helpful in relieving and preventing low backaches and it increases mobility of the lumbar spine and improves the tone of the muscles that control the position and movement of the pelvis.

III. PELVIC ROCKING ON HANDS AND KNEES

Position:

• On hands and knees, hands directly under shoulders.
• Knees directly under hips and about 3–4 inches apart.

Method:

a. Keeping the head in line with the back, tighten the buttocks and lower abdominal muscles, at the same time humping the lower back.
b. Relax the buttocks and lower abdominal muscles, at the same time hollowing the lower back. This rocks the pelvis forward.
c. Repeat the above procedure five or six times in succession.
d. Relax for a few minutes by resting thighs on legs, supporting body on thighs and forehead on crossed arms which rest on floor.

Suggestions and Values:

• This form of pelvic rocking removes pressure from within the pelvis and increases the forward–backward mobility of the pelvis and lumbar spine. It is also helpful in relieving and preventing low backaches.

IV. SQUATTING

Position:

- Stand with feet apart and parallel. The wall may be used as a support (or an open door).

Method:

a. Against the wall, bend knees. Gradually sit down lower and lower until able to sit on heels.
b. Push heels against floor and use big muscles in front of thighs to return to a standing position.
c. Away from wall: take a firm grip on the door knob or heavy piece of furniture. This also may be done with your husband. Stand at arm's length, grasp each other's hands, and proceed with step #4.
d. Squat down with knees *apart* and heels on floor. Do not point toes outward.
e. While sitting on heels bend slightly forward. Raise buttocks, then straighten back, then straighten knees to standing position. Keep back straight. With squatting practice you will find you will get strong enough to squat without holding onto something. Hold position for one minute—no longer.

Suggestions and Value:

a. This exercise promotes slight natural enlargement of pelvis during pregnancy and to stretch the perineum.
b. It will help to prevent muscle soreness after delivery because this is the position assumed on the delivery table.
c. It is useful for reaching low drawers or shelves and for giving attention to the young child. This procedure should also be used when lifting objects from the floor such as a young child, boxes, etc., to prevent low back strain.

V.   KEGAL—TO TEACH CONTROL OF THE PELVIC FLOOR:

• Contract the muscles surrounding the back passage (anus); decontract. Repeat with muscles surrounding the front passages (urethra, vagina) and then the whole pelvic floor. Repeat as often as possible each day.

VI.   ADDUCTOR STRETCHING ISOMETRIC EXERCISE:

• This exercise helps to increase the elasticity of the pelvic floor. Sit on the floor with the soles of your feet together, with heels as close to your body as possible. Place hands under knees with palms up. Pull up against knees with hands and at same time push down against hands with your knees. Hold for 10 seconds.

Breathing Techniques

Introduction: Breathing is designed to correspond to the various stages and phases of labor and delivery. Regular practice of these methods will greatly enhance your effectiveness during the birth process.

BREATHING FOR EARLY LABOR* (FIRST AND SECOND LEVEL BREATHING):

1. Reserved for the time when control is needed.
2. This is the simplest and least tiring of the exercises—so continue as long as possible, as long as it helps—before a more complex breathing is used.

*Contractions are of low to moderate frequency (up to 5 minutes), short duration (30–45 seconds), and low intensity.

3. When practicing this and subsequent exercises, the instructions "CON-TRACTION BEGINS" and then "CONTRACTION ENDS" must be given by the coach or you must mentally instruct yourself.

4. The idea of contraction must be present in order to permit an orderly transition from the exercise as a practice technique to a means of controlling true labor.

5. Since there is a tendency toward drowsiness due to fatigue when in labor, all breathing exercises must be done with the eyes open and fixed on a simple convenient object in the room focal point.

Method:

1. With the command "CONTRACTION BEGINS" inhale deeply through the nose, then exhale completely through the mouth (cleansing breath).

2. Begin slow, deliberate rhythmic chest breathing, inhaling and exhaling through the nose. Achieve a rate of 6 to 9 breaths/minute (first level).

3. When this is mastered, add rhythmic abdominal massage (effleurage) to the technique, performing it simultaneously with the breathing:

   a. with the onset of the contractions, the cupped hands with the fingertips resting on the skin are placed at the lowest point of the abdomen (just above the pubic bone);

   b. while inhaling, stroke the abdomen toward the sides and upward to the level of the umbilicus;

   c. while exhaling, stroke downward in the middle; thus a circular sort of massage is performed;

   d. this should be done simultaneously with the breathing, beginning with the command "CONTRACTION BEGINS" and ending with the command "CONTRACTION ENDS";

   e. to prevent irritation of the skin and hands, talcum powder should be sprinkled liberally on the abdomen during the performance of this exercise.

4. Second level—move your hand up to your lower ribcage, and with your mouth slightly open, breathe in and out, a little less deeply than before. You will notice that your effort now expands the rib cage under your hands rather than concentrating on your diaphragm. Achieve a rate of 16–20 breaths/minute.

BREATHING FOR WELL-ESTABLISHED LABOR
(ACCELERATED)

1. This technique is next in order of complexity to the rhythmic chest breathing.
2. Should be used when the slow breathing becomes ineffective.
3. Technique learned in two stages: first rapid shallow breathing of even rhythm; then, the actual method to be used in labor.
4. Because uterine contractions occur in waves—that is, the intensity begins at a low level, rises to a peak, and then falls off, the rapid shallow breathing should be done in the same fashion, accelerating with the contraction. The rate can be increased to 50–60 breaths per minute.
5. Occasionally some women become slightly dizzy when they first begin to practice this exercise. It is nothing to cause alarm. Tolerance develops quickly, and dizziness disappears.
6. These exercises should be learned in both supine and sitting positions.
7. Most women prefer a modified supine position (with back propped up) during labor, but some prefer to sit.
8. Breathing should now be done in and *out of the mouth.*

BREATHING FOR TRANSITIONAL FIRST STAGE OF LABOR

1. This is the latter phase of the first stage of labor when the following may be observed or felt:
   a. 7–10 cm dilation
   b. Contractions at their peak of frequency, intensity, and duration.
   c. This is more distinct in prima gravida.
2. Exercise designed complex enough and strong enough to overcome the cerebral excitation of transitional contractions and this provides control of this stage of labor—and since it's impossible to push while doing this exercise, it thus overcomes the reflex to do so—until full dilation.
3. For women having second and subsequent children, the exercise is necessary even for the short and poorly defined transition period.

4. When combined with proper pushing and when both are properly used in response to the commands of the doctor, a slow, delicate, and deliberated delivery can be achieved with a minimum of physical assistance.

Exercise:

Method: Pant-blow

- This is a light superficial type of breathing which is punctuated periodically by blowing out and executed according to a particular pattern: Pyramid pant-blow can be modified to include more blowing.
- CONTRACTION BEGINS. Cleansing breath. Rapid light breathing. Blow out. Cleansing breath. CONTRACTION ENDS.
- Practice at least two contractions, each lasting at least 70–90 seconds.

Voluntary Expulsive Efforts (Pushing)

1. Push only on command of obstetrician or nurse—the mother's urge to push and sensation of rectal pressure does not mean the right time for pushing has arrived (full dilation).
2. The lungs are filled with air (this pushed diaphragm down into the abdomen, increasing pressure), the chest is tilted forward and the shoulders rounded slightly (forcing the diaphragm against the abdominal organs), while at the same time the abdominal muscles are powerfully contracted.
3. Along with this pressure it is necessary for simultaneous relaxation of the perineal muscles. This pushing as if it were an open door. Labor has a tendency to close the door, to tighten the muscles of the pelvic floor constricting the vaginal outlet.
4. Training for expulsion has two parts:
   a. learning sufficient control of the muscles of the pelvic floor
   b. controlling and strengthening the abdominal muscles in order to exert proper and sufficient pressure.
5. Practice the actual push for no more than one or two seconds!

Vocabulary

ABDOMEN—belly or stomach
ABORTION—miscarriage; having an early end to pregnancy

ALBUMIN—a protein substance tested for in urine examination

AMNIOTIC FLUID—fluid supporting baby while in uterus

ANEMIA—a condition in which the red corpuscles of the blood are reduced in number, or are deficient in hemoglobin

ANESTHESIA—method for reducing feeling or sensation

ANTEPARTUM—before delivery

ANUS—opening of rectum

BLADDER—organ in which urine collects before voiding

BREECH DELIVERY—delivery of baby with buttocks or feet first

CESAREAN—operation for delivery of baby through abdomen

CATHETERIZATION—emptying of bladder by small tube

CERVIX—lower part of uterus (womb) which opens into the vagina

CIRCUMCISION—removal of foreskin of penis

COLOSTRUM—sticky fluid secreted from nipple of breast during pregnancy and for one or two days after delivery

CONCEPTION—union of sperm and egg, beginning of pregnancy

CONTRACTION—tightening of muscles of uterus

EMBRYO—baby in uterus during first three months of pregnancy

EPISIOTOMY—cut in perineum commonly made to avoid tearing during delivery

FALLOPIAN TUBE—tube through which egg passes from ovary to uterus

FERTILIZATION—see conception

FETAL HEART—baby's heartbeat in uterus

FETUS—baby in uterus

FONTANELS—soft spots on all babies' heads

FORCEPS—instruments occasionally used to aid delivery

FUNDUS—top of uterus

GENITALS—sex organs

HEMORRHOIDS—piles, varicose veins of rectum

INVOLUTION—return of uterus to normal size and condition after delivery

LACERATION—tear

LACTATION—process of producing and supplying milk

LOCHIA—discharge from vagina after delivery

MECONIUM—baby's normal black bowel movement for few days after birth

MEMBRANES—sac or bag lining uterus in which baby grows

MENSTRUAL PERIOD—monthly or period

MUCUS—sticky material found in various discharges

OBSTETRICS—branch of medicine covering care of women in pregnancy, childbirth, and after delivery

OVUM—egg cell

PENIS—male sex organ

PERINEAL CARE—cleansing of external genitals

PERINEUM—tissue surrounding anus and vagina
PLACENTA—afterbirth tissue through which baby is fed while in the uterus, delivered after the baby
POSTPARTUM—after delivery
PREGNANCY—period of time from conception to birth or miscarriage
RECTUM—lower end of the intestines
RUPTURE OF MEMBRANES—breaking of "bag of waters"
SCROTUM—the pouch at the base of the penis containing the testicles
SHOW—blood-tinged mucus discharge
SPERM—male sex cell
STOOL—bowel movement
TERM—usual end of pregnancy
TESTICLE—male organ that produces sperm
TOXEMIA—a medical term for certain complications peculiar to pregnancy
UMBILICAL CORD—cord connecting baby's umbilicus and placenta
URINALYSIS—examination of urine
UTERUS—womb
VAGINA—passage from uterus to outside
VARICOSE VEINS—enlarged or dilated veins
VERNIX CASEOSA—cheese or waxy material covering skin of newborn
VERTEX DELIVERY—delivery of baby with head first
VOIDING—passing of urine

The following are examples of weekly class outlines and handouts given to parents each week.

Class 1

1. Introduction
    A. Who we are.
    B. Who are the teachers.
2. Course Description
    A. What's in this expectant mothers' course?
    B. How will this course help me?
    C. How long will the course last?
    D. When and where will the class meet?
    E. What responsibility do I have in this course?
3. Membership
    A. Who can come?
    B. What are membership cards?

4. Getting to Know Each Other
   A. Refreshments.
   B. Mingling and having fun.

Class 2

Nutrition

1. What is nutrition?

2. Why is nutrition important to me and my growing fetus?

3. How does my baby (fetus) "eat"?

4. Why is nutrition especially important for teenagers who are pregnant?

5. What can happen if I don't feed my baby (fetus) the foods he/she needs?

6. Filling out nutrition questionnaire.

Class 3

Early Pregnancy

1. I'm pregnant. What now?

2. What changes will I have to make?

3. Who can help me?

Conception

1. What is conception?

2. Why don't I have a menstrual period when I am pregnant?

3. Exactly where in me is my baby (fetus)?

4. How big is the baby (fetus) at first? How fast does he grow?

5. What can he do inside of me?

Class 4

Knowing My Body

1. What and where are my three external pelvic openings?

2. How do my organs inside shift to make room for my baby?

3. What are my female sex organs?

4. How does the doctor make a vaginal examination?

Physical Changes During Pregnancy

1. Why do I have to urinate so often?

2. Why do I *now* have a constipation problem? Will anything help?

3. Is heartburn normal? What can I do about this problem?

4. Why do I pass so much gas?

5. What are the new marks on my stomach? Will they go away?

6. Why are my breasts getting bigger? Will they stay this way?

Class 5

Labor and Delivery

1. What things have I heard about labor and delivery?

2. When do I know I am in true labor?

3. What should I do?

4. What happens to me when I get to the hospital?

5. What will happen to me during labor?
   5.1 Stages of labor

6. How will the classes, exercises, and breathing techniques help me during labor and delivery?

7. Do I need medication for pain during labor? What kind might I receive? What will the medication do?

Class 6

Complications

1. What is toxemia and how is it harmful?

2. How do anemias affect me and my baby?

3. What are urinary tract infections?

4. If I get German measles while I'm pregnant, can they hurt my baby?

5. Can VD or GC hurt my baby?

6. What is Rh factor and what does it mean?

7. Why do miscarriages occur?

8. What about birth defects?

Class 7

Breast Feeding and Bottle Feeding

1. What are the advantages of breast feeding?

2. What are the advantages of bottle feeding?

3. How do I take care of my breasts during pregnancy and during nursing?

4. How to succeed at breast feeding.

5. How can I breast feed if I want to go back to school or to work?

6. Preparing baby's bottles and sterilizing formula.

7. Why is close contact with my baby so important during feeding?

8. What about vitamins?

Class 8

Knowing My Baby

Infant Bonding

1. What will my baby be like?

2. How will life be different after my baby comes?

    2.1. How can I continue important activities in my life?

3. Do all new mothers automatically "feel" like mothers?

4. How to have a close relationship with my baby.

5. Is it normal to have angry and resentful feelings toward my baby?

6. How to share the care of baby and still maintain responsibility for the baby myself.

7. How do you feel when relatives, neighbors, and strangers tell you that you're doing something wrong?

Class 9

Family Planning

1. Why do people plan their future families?

2. What are the advantages of planning or spacing your children?

3. What are the ways available to me to prevent unwanted pregnancies?

4. What are the consequences of having babies too close together?

PART TWO
PARENTING CLASSES AND HANDOUTS

Schedule

Introduction

OBJECTIVES

a. To help you develop an awareness of the ways that your baby grows and learns to cope with his/her world.
b. To promote better understanding and more skillful appreciation of good infant–child care.
c. To assist you in meeting and overcoming problems that arise from having a growing, ever-changing baby in the family.
d. To help you maintain your baby in optimum health through the teaching of good health care, periodic physical exams, and maintenance of immunization schedule.
e. To share your child-rearing experience with other mothers with babies in the same age groups.

1. What are some of the new situations you are faced with now that the baby is awake for longer periods and has become more active?
2. What makes your baby fussy or irritable now that he's older, that didn't make any difference before?
3. What hazards to the baby must you watch for that weren't apparent before?
4. What games does your baby like to play with you and others close to the family?
5. How does your baby amuse himself/herself when left alone?

A New View of Baby's World—Behavior and Emotional Norms, 4–8 mos.

EMOTIONAL DEVELOPMENT:

What is the first developmental need of an infant?

Through what processes is this need developed?

Who helps the baby develop this? How?

How is mistrust learned?

SOCIAL DEVELOPMENT:

In early infancy, a baby is basically passive. What are the first social responses that a mother notices in her baby?

As the baby reaches 3–4 months, what are his or her new responses to the mother or caretaker?

Name some of the frustrations a 4–6 month infant may face.

What determines how the baby will handle these conflicts or frustrations?

> The sense of trust is the cornerstone of a wholesome personality. Either a harmonious relationship of giving and getting is established or disruption occurs and other modes of behavior predominate in the infant, such as feeding difficulties and excessive crying. Instead of mutual satisfaction there is mutual frustration between mother and infant.
>
> *Marlow*

Mothering Class Schedule

OBJECTIVES

1. To help you develop an awareness of the ways that your Baby grows and learns to cope with his world.
2. To provide additional training in infant care.
3. To assist you in overcoming problems that arise from having a new baby in the family.
4. To help you maintain your baby in optimum health through the teaching of good health care, periodic physical exams, and maintenance of immunization schedule.
5. To share your experiences with other new mothers.

    I. Infant's daily routine—Feeding, Bathing
   II. Growth and development—knowing your baby
  III. Safety—at home and in the car; child abuse
  IV. How to communicate with your baby.
   V. Planning for you and your baby's future.
  VI. Introduction to solid foods.
 VII. Physical restoration of mother.
VIII. When is your baby sick—preventative measures—temperature taking
  IX. Growth and development—age of appropriate games and playing with baby
   X. Evaluation and open discussion of client-selected topics

FEEDING—BATHING—INFANT'S DAILY ROUTINE

A. Breast Feeding—How does it fit into my life?

B. Formula Feeding—Why are cleanliness and boiling important?

C. Spoon Feeding—Why use a spoon for solid foods such as cereal?

D. Bathing—Why is a daily bath important?
   1. Cleanliness
   2. Playing
   3. Exercising
   4. Inspecting baby's body
   5. Communicating

E. Daily Routine—Why is "scheduling" important to you and the baby?

Knowing Your Baby

What can my baby do now?

What will he do next?

Are his accomplishments normal for age?

How can I keep him from getting hurt?

1. falling
2. suffocation
3. drowning
4. auto travel
5. electrical shock

6. burns
7. too rough play

> All parents feel incompetent and despairing at times when they are unable to understand the child's cues and to meet his needs, but if self-confidence is constantly lacking, the parents' despair may turn to anger, rejection and abuse.

Safety for Infant and Child

What are the hazards to my baby in the first year?

What safety measures should I take?

What else can I do to prevent injury or death to my baby?

What is child abuse?

When and where is it found?

What are some of the causes?

QUIZ

1. At what age do you think most babies can sit alone?
2. What vitamins do we need to add to an infant diet?

3. Should a baby be more warmly dressed than an adult?
4. How many shots are needed to prevent measles?
5. If a mother is nervous and tense or angry and upset, when she is handling the baby, would it change the way the baby acts?
6. At what age can a baby wriggle and roll off a table or bed?
7. What position, or place, in a car is the most safe for a baby? most dangerous?

How Does My Baby Communicate With Me?

A. What does my baby's cry mean?
   1. How can I tell the difference from one cry to another?

B. How else does my baby talk with me?

C. How can I help my baby learn to talk?

D. What games do babies like to play?

   • How do they help baby to learn?
   • What do they teach baby?

The child needs to feel his behavior will produce an effect or he will stop contacting his parents.

Planning For You And Your Baby's Future

Why do people plan the size of their family?

What are the advantages of "wanted" pregnancies?

What ways are there to keep from having babies?

Why is it more a risk for teenagers to have babies?

How does having a baby especially affect a teenager's way of life?

The parents may want a baby but be dismayed to discover that he is not like their expectations.

Introduction of Solid Foods

Why give a baby under one year of age solid food?

What age do parents usually start solid foods?

What benefits does the baby get from solid food?

What are the disadvantages of starting solid foods early?

Which method of feeding solid foods is preferred?

A mother holding and talking to baby while feeding conveys satisfaction and security to her infant.

Food means more than nourishment to the baby; it is his early contact with the outside world and his first step toward independence.

Physical Restoration of Mother

Why do I tire so easily?

What can I do to help me feel and look my best?

What exercises can I do to get my figure back?

1. abdominal
2. waist
3. arms and chest
4. buttocks and thighs
5. general muscular tone

When Is My Baby Sick?

How can I tell when my baby is sick? What do I look for?

How can I tell if my baby has a fever?
How do I read a thermometer?

What do I have to watch most carefully in a newborn?

_____ in a 1- to 3-month-old baby?

_____ in a 3- to 6-month-old baby?

Is it alright to toss a baby around when playing?

What's croup?
How do I handle it?

What is colic?
How can I help my baby through it?

What "shots" are given to the baby for protection from disease?
When?
How often?

Growth and Development

1. How does a baby grow?

2. In what ways do babies differ in growth and development?

3. How does the rate of development change in the first year?

4. What is the order in growth?
   (What comes first, second——last?)

5. How does the home environment affect growth and development?

6. What dreams do you have for the fullest possible development for your children?

7. How much can you help your baby accomplish these?

Mothering Classes: Evaluation

Leader:

Please help me to make this a more meaningful experience for you by answering the following questions. Thank you.

1. What did you hope to get out of these sessions?

2. What did you actually get out of these sessions?

3. What did you like best about these sessions?

4. What did you like least about these sessions?

5. What was most important to you? Please number in order of importance with #1 being most important.
   ___ Learning about baby care
   ___ Learning how baby grows and develops
   ___ Learning to play with baby
   ___ Learning how to be a better parent
   ___ Getting together with other new mothers
   ___ Learning how to prevent accidents and illness of baby

6. How would you change these sessions?

7. Would you like to bring other new mothers and babies to these sessions?

8. Do you feel these sessions have helped you? In what way?

9. In the next series of meetings, which topics would be of most interest to you? List in order of importance with #1 being most important.
   ___ Baby's behavior development
   ___ Baby's emotional development
   ___ Your future in the career world
   ___ Sleep problems of your baby
   ___ Safety of baby now that he or she is moving about
   ___ Growth and development from 4–8 months
   ___ Feeding (vitamins, solid foods, weaning)
   ___ Your feelings about being a mother
   ___ Babysitters and nursery schools
   ___ Others (give suggestions)
10. What other activities would you like to see started at these sessions?

Prepared Childbirth Teaching Outline (Couples Classes)

R. COLOMBO, RN, BS

M. NEWTON, RN

S. GIBSON, RN

S. ANGERMEIER, RN
All are childbirth educators with St. Anthony's Hospital in St. Petersburg, Fl.

PART ONE
ST. ANTHONY'S HOSPITAL, INC.
PREPARED CHILDBIRTH CLASS OUTLINE

I. TARGET POPULATION

The client is defined as a gravid female and her significant other.

A. The clients have previously attended a series of basic family-centered maternity classes.
B. The client is in the third trimester of pregnancy.
C. The client's medical doctor or midwife is aware that she is attending the prepared childbirth class.
D. The clients are planning to deliver in a hospital setting.
E. The clients are of childbearing age.

II. LEARNING NEEDS AND RATIONALE

A. The client needs to learn that the process of labor should be a positive experience for both participants.

   Pregnant women fear physical damage during childbirth and these fears exist at an unconscious level.[1]

B. The client needs to learn that labor is a predictable process.

   The woman knows that she will have no part in determining when this threatening event will occur. For this reason, the element of control or lack of it can assume great importance. According to Peplau, nursing is, ". . . a therapeutic intervention which enables the patient to incorporate past experience into the continuum of their total experience."[2]

C. The client needs knowledge of pelvic anatomy and its physiology during labor.

According to Gagne, stimulus response connection and verbal association are prerequisite to the learning of concepts, principles, and problem solving. Gagne RM: *The Conditions of Learning.* New York, Holt, Rinehart and Winston, 1965.

D. The client–couple should learn to enhance their ability to communicate their needs to each other using nonverbal communication.

   "As she (the pregnant woman) enters the third trimester . . . time and identity take on a new significance for her in a new sense of alienation and uncertainty for what is real and what is unreal." Touch interrupts this sea of alienation, of isolation, and provides the means for reality orientation.[3]

E. The client needs to learn and apply the mechanics of conscious relaxation.

1. Cassidy JE: A Nurse Looks at Childbirth Anxiety, *JOGN,* Jan/Feb 1974, p. 52.
2. *Ibid.* p. 53.
3. Rubin R: Cognitive Style in Pregnancy, *AJN,* March 1970, p. 508.

According to Dick-Read, perception of pain can be intensified when the parturient falls victim to the fear–tension–pain syndrome.[4]

F. The coach–client needs to learn his/her role during labor as being one of care, comfort, and communication.

Previously, fatherhood had been looked upon as a social obligation with no biological or instructive roots for fatherliness. It was defined merely as the human male role in procreation.[5]

III. COURSE DESCRIPTION

The prepared childbirth program is a series of four classes. These classes provide a foundation for the client (pregnant woman and her significant other) to have a positive experience in participating in the delivery of their child through the use of breathing and relaxation technique. Concepts of normal physiology are explored and possible complications or unknown factors that may develop during labor are also explained.

IV. GOAL STATEMENT

The couple will attend a series of four classes in prepared childbirth during which they will learn to utilize conscious relaxation, breathing exercises, and comfort measures for use during labor and delivery. The couple will explore means of coping with unforeseen problems of labor and delivery.

4. Dick-Read G: *Childbirth Without Fear.* New York, Harper & Row, 1970.
5. Gollober M: A Comment on the Need for Father-Infant Interaction, *JOGN*, Sep/Oct 1976, p. 18.

V.   COURSE OBJECTIVES

By the completion of this course in prepared childbirth, the clients will:

A. Generalize about the physiologic changes occurring within the pregnant woman during the third trimester.
B. Describe the discomforts often encountered in late pregnancy and during labor, their causes, and the measures that may alleviate them.
C. Predict the functions and course of labor.
D. Traverse their childbearing experience with a minimum of anxiety.
E. Discuss factors that will influence the ease with which they will make the personal transition into parenthood. Such factors are personal and societal expectations, capabilities, and limitations.
F. Enhance their relationship with the unborn family member.
G. Establish a relationship with other couples who are undergoing the maturational crisis of childbearing.
H. Prepare a groundwork of knowledge and skills upon which to base more advanced information to be encountered in the fourth trimester.

PART TWO
COURSE OUTLINE

CLASS ONE

1.0 Objective

By the end of this class, the client will perform the following physical conditioning exercises at least 3 times:

- Tailor reach
- Tailor press
- Kegal
- Leg raises

1.1 Teaching Strategies

The instructor will:

1.1.1 distribute and review the booklet *Preparation for Childbearing*
1.1.2 explain the rationale for each exercise
1.1.3 demonstrate the exercises as illustrated in the above booklet
1.1.4 explain the use of the homework sheet
1.1.5 answer questions

1.2 Criteria for Evaluation

The client will:

1.2.1 return the demonstration in class
1.2.2 consistently complete the homework sheet in the following weeks
1.2.3 state on the postdelivery evaluation form that they have practiced body-conditioning at home

2.0 By the end of this class the client–couple will demonstrate these positions of comfort illustrated in the *Preparation for Childbearing* booklet:

- side-lying
- supine
- rising from the bed

2.1 Teaching Strategies

The instructor will:

2.1.1 explain rationale for each position
2.1.2 ask the coach to place client in each position

2.2 Criteria for Evaluation

The client will:

2.2.1 demonstrate each position correctly

2.2.2 subsequently utilize these positions as a conditioned response when appropriate

2.2.3 state on the postdelivery evaluation form that they have practiced positions of comfort at home

3.0 By the end of this class, the client will cite at least one comfort measure for each of the following discomforts of pregnancy:

- leg cramps
- back pain
- heartburn
- nocturia
- shortness of breath
- round ligament pain

3.1 Teaching Strategies

The instructor will:

3.1.1 assess client's knowledge of comfort measures

3.1.2 explain cause of discomfort

3.1.3 enumerate several comfort measures for each discomfort

4.0 By the end of this class, the client will demonstrate the technique of conscious relaxation for application during labor.

4.1 Teaching Strategies

The instructor will:

4.1.1 explain principles of conscious relaxation

4.1.2   using coach as a model, demonstrate the process of conscious relaxation

4.1.2.2   place coach in supine position with knees supported

4.1.2.3   use a focal point

4.1.2.4   instruct the coach to contract and relax alternately specific muscles on command

4.1.3   repeat the above process, replacing the coach with the expectant mother

4.2   Criteria for Evaluation

The client will:

4.2.1   during the span of the four classes, demonstrate with progressive improvement the technique of conscious relaxation

4.2.2   apply conscious relaxation technique as a conditioned response during process of labor

4.2.3   state on the postdelivery evaluation form that they have practiced conscious relaxation technique at home

5.0   By the end of this class, the client will identify from a chart:
vagina, uterus, bladder, rectum, cervix, symphysis pubis, sacral prominence, urethra, placenta, cord, membranes, mucous plug, perineum

5.1   Teaching Strategy

The instructor will:

5.1.1   assess the client's ability to name the pelvic and placental parts

5.1.2   indicate the positions and relationships of these body parts using the Birth Atlas

5.1.3   answer questions

5.2   Criteria for Evaluation

The client will:

5.2.1   be able to identify pelvic and placental parts from Birth Atlas

5.2.2 Utilize appropriate anatomical terminology when discussing their concepts in the class

6.0 By the end of this class the client will name three signs of impending labor and respond to each with appropriate behavior.

6.1   Teaching Strategies

The instructor will:

6.1.1 assess the client's knowledge of signs of impending labor
6.1.2 list on the blackboard five signs of impending labor
6.1.3 utilize the Birth Atlas to explain the physiology of each sign
6.1.4 describe behavior appropriate for each of the five signs of impending labor

6.2   Criteria for Evaluation

The client will:

6.2.1 correctly name three signs of impending labor
6.2.2 during rehearsal of labor match appropriate behavior with each of the signs of impending labor

7.0 By the end of this class, the client will describe the physiology of the latent phase of the first stages of labor.

7.1   Teaching Strategies

The instructor will:

7.1.1 define effacement, dilatation, contraction and relate these terms to the latent phase of labor
7.1.2 illustrate the effect of uterine contractions on cervical dilatation and effacement, using knitted uterus and Ross cervical dilatation chart

7.2   Criteria for Evaluation

The client will:

7.2.1 utilize the terms dilatation, effacement, and contraction appropriately when discussing concepts related to the latent phase

7.2.2 when asked during the rehearsal of labor, in Class 4, describe physiology of the latent phase of the first stage of labor

8.0   By the end of this class, the client will describe the emotions of the mother during the latent phase of the first stage of the labor.

8.1   Teaching Strategies

The instructor will:

8.1.1 assess the client's concept of the emotions experienced during latent phase of labor

8.1.2 delineate emotions commonly felt during latent phase

8.2   Criteria for Evaluation

The client will:

8.2.1 describe two emotions commonly felt during latent phase

8.2.2 match the emotions experienced by the mother to her behavior in the latent phase of the first stage labor, when asked during the labor rehearsal, Class 4

9.0   By the end of this class the client will relate the coaching and supportive measures used by the coach to the feelings of the mother during the latent phase of the first stage of labor.

9.1   Teaching Strategies

The instructor will:

9.1.1 restate emotions of mother

9.1.2 state coaching measures such as timing contractions, diversional activity, and moral support

9.1.3 acquaint client with pages 38–39 in *Preparation for Childbearing* as reference

9.2 Criteria for Evaluation

The coach will:

9.2.1 name described coaching measures such as timing contractions, diversional activity, and moral support

9.2.2 intergrate coaching and supportive measures appropriate to the feelings of the mother during the latent phase of the first stage of labor, demonstrate during the practice labor session in Class 4

10.0 By the end of this class, the client will demonstrate slow chest breathing as follows:

—8–12 breaths per minute
—deep cleansing breath at beginning and end of contraction
—concomitant relaxation
—practice for 60 seconds
—concomitant effleurage

10.1 Teaching Strategies

The instructor will:

10.1.1 explain rationale for slow-chest breathing

10.1.2 stress importance of using conscious relaxation while performing slow-chest breathing technique

10.1.3 demonstrate slow-chest breathing

10.1.4 place client in supine position with knees supported by pillow and head elevated

10.1.5 ask client to demonstrate slow-chest breathing technique

10.2   Criteria for Evaluation

The client will:

10.2.1 discuss benefits of slow-chest breathing

10.2.2 demonstrate slow-chest breathing correctly incorporating into technique:

—8–12 breaths per minute

—deep cleansing breath at beginning and end of contraction

—concomitant relaxation

—practice for 60 seconds

—concomitant effleurage

10.2.3 state on the postdelivery evaluation form that they have practiced slow-chest breathing at home

CLASS TWO

1.0   Objective

By the end of this class, the clients will review the content of the previous class.

1.1   Teaching Strategies

The instructor will:

1.1.1 assess client's knowledge of comfort measures, physiology of latent phase of first stage of labor, emotions of mother, and coaching and supporting measures

1.1.2 utilize Birth Atlas, knitted uterus, or labor graph to dispel misconceptions clients may have on labor

1.1.3 evaluate client's technique in demonstrating slow-chest breathing

1.2   Criteria for Evaluation

The client will:

1.2.1   summarize correctly aspects of labor related to the latent phase of the first stage of labor

1.2.2   demonstrate correctly slow-chest breathing and apply this knowledge to labor process

2.0   Objective

By the end of this class the client will describe the physiology of the active phase of the first stage of labor.

2.1   Teaching Strategies

The instructor will:

2.1.1   review terms of effacement, dilation, and uterine contractions and relate these to the active phase of labor

2.1.2   illustrate the effect of uterine contractions on cervical dilation and effacement, using knitted uterus and Ross cervical dilation chart

2.1.3   contrast quality of active phase contractions to latent phase contractions by sketching on blackboard

2.2   Criteria for Evaluation

The client will:

2.2.1   utilize the terms dilation, effacement, and contraction appropriately when discussing concepts related to active phase

2.2.2   when asked during rehearsal of labor in class, describe physiology of active phase of first stage of labor

3.0   Objective

By the end of this class, the client will describe the feelings of the mother during the active phase of the first stage of labor.

3.1 Teaching Strategies

The instructor will:

3.1.1 assess the client's concept of the emotions experienced during the active phase

3.1.2 delineate emotions commonly felt during active phase such as growing serious, apprehension, doubt, increasing introversion, and preoccupation to bodily sensations

3.2 Criteria for Evaluation

The client will:

3.2.1 describe four emotions commonly felt during active phase

3.2.2 when asked during the rehearsal of labor in Class 4, relate the emotions experienced by the mother to her behavior

4.0 Objective

By the end of this class, the client will relate the coaching and supportive measures used by the coach to the feelings of the mother during the active phase of the first stage of labor.

4.1 Teaching Strategies

The instructor will:

4.1.1 restate emotions of mother

4.1.2 state coaching measures such as subdued environment, reassurance, empty bladder, back pressure, verbal and nonverbal moral support, and wet mouth

4.1.3 acquaint client with pages 38–39 in *Preparation for Childbearing* as reference

4.2 Criteria for Evaluation

The coach will:

4.2.1 name described coaching measures such as subdued environment, reassurance, empty bladder, back pressure, and encourage moral support and wet mouth

4.2.2 intergrate coaching and supportive measures appropriate to the feelings of the mother during the active phase of the first stage of labor, demonstrable during practice session in Class 4

5.0 Objective

By the end of this class, the client will demonstrate accelerated–decelerated breathing as follows:

—deep cleansing breath at beginning and end

—shallow breaths, increasing during increment and decreasing during decrement of each contraction

—concomitant relaxation and effleurage

—practice for 60 seconds

5.1 Teaching Strategies

5.1.1 explain rationale for accelerated–decelerated breathing

5.1.2 stress importance of using conscious relaxation and focal point while performing accelerated–decelerated breathing technique

5.1.3 demonstrate accelerated–decelerated breathing

5.1.4 place client in side relaxation position with pillow between knees and under abdomen

5.1.5 utilize thigh squeeze as a simulated contraction on second practice

5.1.6 ask client to return demonstration of the accelerated–decelerated breathing technique

5.2 Criteria for Evaluation

The client will:

5.2.1 discuss benefits of accelerated–decelerated breathing

5.2.2 demonstrate accelerated–decelerated breathing correctly incorporating into technique

    —deep cleansing breath at beginning and end
    —shallow breaths, increasing during increment and decrement of each contraction
    —concomitant relaxation and effleurage
    —practice for 60 seconds

5.2.3 state on postdelivery evaluation form that they have practiced accelerated and decelerated breathing

6.0 Objective

By the end of this class, the clients will contrast the use of analgesia and anesthesia.

6.1 Teaching Strategies

The instructor will:

6.1.1 define terms analgesia and anesthesia

6.1.2 assess client's knowledge of analgesia and anesthesia

6.1.3 list on blackboard names of analgesic drugs used in labor, type of medication, route of administration, and effects on client

6.1.4 differentiate types of anesthesia and, utilizing Ross flip chart, indicate method of administration and effect on client

6.2 Criteria for Evaluation

The client will:

6.2.1 use terms analgesia and anesthesia appropriately and relate their use during the labor and delivery

6.2.2 state on postdelivery evaluation form that they understood types of analgesia and anesthesia available to them

6.2.3 during the rehearsal of labor in Class 4, if asked, discuss effects of medication on client

7.0 Objective

By the end of this class, the client will state the rationale and methods of induction.

7.1 Teaching Strategies

The instructor will:

7.1.1 define induction and its ramifications
7.1.2 differentiate between medically indicated induction and elective induction
7.1.3 describe procedure for induction as follows
   —medication used—oxytoxin and its effect on contraction
   —equipment used such as IV pump, fetal monitor
   —physical preparations
7.1.4 answer questions

7.2 Criteria of Evaluation

The client will:

7.2.1 use term induction correctly and state rationale for use of each
7.2.2 predict the effect of oxytoxin induction on the strength and frequency of contractions
7.2.3 when asked, in rehearsal for labor session in Class 4, discuss induction of labor procedure

8.0 Objective

By the end of this class, the client will relate hospital policy and procedures that apply to the labor and delivery experience.

8.1 Teaching Strategies

The instructor will:

8.1.1 integrate hospital policy and procedure with a tour of the obstetrical department indicating the following:

—labor room: location, equipment used in procedures, mechanics of bed, location of bathroom

—lounge area: location, bathroom, locker for change to scrub suit

—delivery room: where coach sits; equipment and routine

—recovery room: equipment and length of stay

—nursery: routine for newborns

—postpartum: routine, equipment in room

8.1.2 answer questions

8.2 Criteria for Evaluation

The client will:

8.2.1 on admission to the hospital demonstrate his/her ability to find his way about the unit (familiar surroundings) with a minimal asking of questions; this in contrast to the unprepared couple

CLASS THREE

1.0 Objective

By the end of this class the client will review the content of the previous class.

1.1 Teaching Strategies

The instructor will:

1.1.1 assess the client's knowledge of the physiology of the active phase of labor, emotions of the mother, and coaching and supportive measures during the active phase, analgesia, anesthesia, and hospital policy

1.1.2 evaluate the client's technique in demonstrating accelerated–decelerated breathing

1.1.3 answer questions

1.2 Criteria

The client will:

1.2.1 correctly summarize progress during the active phase of the first stage of labor

1.2.2 demonstrate correctly accelerated–decelerated breathing and apply this breathing technique with the knowledge of the labor process

2.0 Objective

By the end of this class, the client will describe the physiology of the transitional phase of the first stage of labor.

2.1 Teaching Strategies

The instructor will:

2.1.1 review terms of effacement, dilatation, uterine contractions, and station, and relate this to the transitional phase of labor

2.1.2 contrast the quality, frequency, and duration of the transitional phase contractions with the previous two phases

2.1.3 illustrate, using the knitted uterus and bony pelvis, the progressive effect of uterine contractions on the descent of the head

2.1.4 relate the position of the infant's head to urge to push

2.2 Criteria

The client will:

2.2.1 utilize the terms dilatation, effacement, contraction, station, and position appropriately when discussing concepts related to the transitional phase

2.2.2 when asked during the rehearsal of labor in Class 4, describe the physiology of the active phase of the first stage of labor

3.0   Objective

By the end of this class the client will describe the feelings of the mother during the transitional phase of the first stage of labor.

3.1   Teaching Strategies

The instructor will:

3.1.1 assess the clients' concept of the emotions experienced during the transitional phase

3.1.2 delineate the emotions commonly felt during the active phase such as panic, irritability, desire to quit, short attention span

3.2   Criteria

The client will:

3.2.1 describe two emotions commonly felt during the transitional phase

3.2.2 when asked during rehearsal of labor in Class 4, relate the emotions experienced by the mother to her behavior

4.0   Objective

By the end of this class, the client will relate the coaching and supportive measures used by the coach to the feelings of the mother during the transitional phase of the first stage of labor.

4.1   Teaching Strategies

The instructor will:

4.1.1 restate emotions of mother

4.1.2 state coaching measures, such as using instrumental language, breathing with parturient, using eyes as focal point, notifying parturient of beginning of contraction (if she has been medicated), respecting parturient's possible need not to be touched

4.1.3 enumerate possible physical discomforts experienced by mother such as diaphoresis, nausea and/or vomiting, leg trembling

4.1.4 acquaint client with pages 38–39 in *Preparation For Childbearing* as reference

4.2 Criteria

The coach will:

4.2.1 when asked, describe the coaching measures appropriate for the situation

4.2.2 integrate coaching and supportive measures appropriate to feelings of the mother during the fourth class rehearsal for labor

5.0 Objective

By the end of this class, the client will demonstrate pant-blow breathing as follows:

—deep cleansing breath at the beginning and end of each contraction

—at least three shallow pants interrupted with a blow

—blowing continuously if there is an urge to push

—concomitant relaxation

—practice 90 seconds

5.1 Teaching Strategies

The instructor will:

5.1.1 place client in Tailor sit position

5.1.2 explain the rationale of pant-blow breathing

5.1.3 stress the necessity of avoiding the urge to push by blowing

5.1.4 stress the importance of using conscious relaxation and a focal point while performing pant-blow breathing

5.1.5 demonstrate pant-blow breathing

5.1.6 ask client to return the demonstration

5.2 Criteria

The client will:

5.2.1 discuss the benefits of pant-blow breathing

5.2.2 demonstrate pant-blow breathing correctly, incorporating into the technique:

—deep cleansing breath at the beginning and end of each contraction

—at least three shallow pants interrupted with a blow

—blowing continuously if there is an urge to push

—concomitant relaxation

—practice for 90 seconds

5.2.3 state on the postdelivery evaluation form that they have practiced pant-blow breathing

6.0 Objective

By the end of this class, the client will predict how they will handle less than ideal situations such as third trimester bleeding, prolonged labor, fetal heart tone irregularities, delivery under general anesthesia, and abnormalities of the newborn.

6.1 Teaching Strategies

The instructor will:

6.1.1 open discussion concerning topics pertaining to their labor which clients may fear

6.1.2 relate to the client the normalcy of these fears

6.1.3 clarify and correct any unfounded fears

6.1.4 encourage the clients to discuss how they would react in such a situation

6.1.5 encourage the clients to continue this discussion with each other at home, playing the game "What if . . ." and exchanging expectations that they would hold for themselves and for each other

6.2   Criteria

The client will:

6.2.1   participate in group discussion, if only nonverbally, in class

6.2.2   report in the rehearsal for labor in the fourth class how they believe they would react to untoward situations

7.0   Objective

By the end of this class, the client will report indications for Cesarean section, additional preparation for it, and general information regarding recovery from a Cesarean section.

7.1   Teaching Strategies

The instructor will:

7.1.1   review procedures in Obstetrical Department concerning Cesarean section prior to class

7.1.2   assess client's knowledge of a Cesarean section and what this term means to them

7.1.3   describe indications for a Cesarean section and give rationale for why it is done

7.1.4   contrast preparation for a Cesarean section with a vaginal delivery as follows:

—explanation of need for a Cesarean section

—abdominal vaginal prep

—Foley catheter in bladder

—medications used

7.1.5   differentiate recovery from a Cesarean section versus vaginal delivery as follows

—stay in recovery room is three hours

—abdominal incision covered by a dressing

—postoperative pain relieved by medication

—slow-chest breathing and concomitant relaxation

—hospital stay approximately five to six days

—longer recuperation period at home

7.1.6 discuss postpartum phase of recovery period as follows:
  —care of incision
  —vaginal lochia present
  —breast care
  —fundus of uterus check
  —instruction on infant care, self-care, and adaptation of family members to the new infant
7.1.7 integrate this information during all four classes of the Prepared Childbirth Program

7.2 Criteria

The client will:

7.2.1 use term Cesarean section appropriately and state three indications for why it may be performed
7.2.2 name two procedures done prior to Cesarean section not done before vaginal delivery
7.2.3 discuss three ways a recovery period from a Cesarean section differs from a vaginal delivery
7.2.4 when asked, in rehearsal of labor session in class 4, discuss implications of Cesarean section delivery

CLASS FOUR

1.0 Objective

By the end of this class, the client will describe the physiology of the second stage of labor.

1.1 Teaching Strategies

The instructor will:

1.1.1 review terms effacement, dilatation, and uterine contractions and relate this to the second stage of labor

1.1.2 contrast the quality, frequency, and duration of expulsive phase contractions with the previous phases

1.1.3 illustrate the progressive effect of uterine contractions on the descent of the baby's head using the knitted uterus and bony pelvis

1.2   Criteria

The client will:

1.2.1 utilize terms dilatation, effacement, contraction, station, and position appropriately when discussing concepts related to expulsive phase

1.2.2 when asked during rehearsal of labor, describe physiology of expulsive phase

2.0   Objective

By the end of this class, the client will describe the feelings of the mother during the second stage of labor.

2.1   Teaching Strategies

The instructor will:

2.1.1 assess client's concept of emotions experienced during expulsive phase of labor

2.1.2 delineate emotions commonly felt during expulsive phase such as relief, pleased to be able to take active part, attentive about pushing, more alert, and a spurt of energy

2.2   Criteria

The client will:

2.2.1 describe two emotions commonly felt during expulsive phase of labor

2.2.2 when asked during rehearsal of labor, relate emotions experienced by the mother

3.0 Objective

By the end of this class, the client will relate the coaching and supportive measures used by the coach to the feelings of the mother during the second stage of labor.

3.1 Teaching Strategies

Instructor will:

3.1.1 restate emotions of mother

3.1.2 state coaching measures such as prop-up in bed, encourage to relax between contractions, reassurance, guidance in pushing with each contraction

3.1.3 acquaint client with pages 38–39 in *Preparation For Childbearing* booklet for reference

3.2 Criteria

Client will:

3.2.1 when asked, describe coaching measures appropriate for the situation

3.2.2 integrate coaching and supportive measures apropos to feelings of mother during rehearsal labor

4.0 Objective

By the end of this class, the client will demonstrate the breathing pattern for the expulsive phase of labor as follows:

—begin with one deep cleansing breath

—take a second deep breath and hold throughout contraction

—if a third breath is necessary before the end of the contraction, repeat the second step

4.1   Teaching Strategies

The instructor will:

4.1.1 explain rationale of breathing technique

4.1.2 place client in semi-Fowler's position with back supported by coach and pillows

4.1.3 demonstrate the technique as follows
   —cleansing breath as contraction begins
   —draw legs to side of abdomen, holding thighs, ankles, or feet
   —take second deep breath and hold
   —flex chin on chest, bearing down in direction of pelvic outlet
   —hold as long as possible
   —if third breath is necessary before end of contraction, take a deep breath and hold
   —cleansing breath at end of contraction

4.2   Criteria

The client will:

4.2.1 correctly demonstrate expulsive phase breathing pattern
   —begin with one deep cleansing breath
   —take a second deep breath and hold throughout contraction
   —if a third breath is necessary before the end of the contraction, repeat the second step

4.2.2 state on the postdelivery form that they have practiced expulsive phase breathing

5.0   Objective

By the end of this class, the client will describe the routine procedures in the delivery room in preparation for the birth of the baby

5.1   Teaching Strategies

The instructor will:

5.1.1 state at which point the laboring mother may be brought to the delivery room

5.1.2 list physical preparation of mother as follows:
—lithotomy position
—Betadine skin prep
—draping with sterile sheets
—administration of pudendal block
—episiotomy performed
5.1.3 describe typical characteristics of the newborn and its immediate care

5.2 Criteria

The client will:

5.2.1 predict course of events in the delivery room
5.2.2 when asked, describe the normal newborn

6.0 Objective

By the end of this class, the client will identify the mechanics of the third stage of labor.

6.1 Teaching Strategies

The instructor will:

6.1.1 assess the clients' knowledge of feelings of participants immediately after delivery of baby
6.1.2 review briefly function of the placenta
6.1.3 review physiology of expulsion of the placenta by using the birth atlas
6.1.4 discuss medications given to mother at this time
6.1.5 outline mother's role in expulsion of placenta

6.2 Criteria

The client will:

6.2.1 identify placenta on birth atlas and describe its function
6.2.2 predict mother's role during expulsion of placenta

7.0 Objective

By the end of this class, the client will discuss with the instructor the advantages of family-centered maternity care and how mother–baby coupling will enhance their relationship with the newborn.

7.1 Teaching Strategies

The instructor will:

7.1.1 review literature on family-centered maternity care and mother–baby coupling

7.1.2 review the policies and procedures of St. Anthony's maternity unit

7.1.3 introduce the concepts of family-centered maternity and mother–baby coupling

7.1.4 describe how the father's participation in labor and delivery, unlimited visiting, and modified rooming-in is implemented at St. Anthony's

7.1.5 answer questions

7.2 Criteria

The client will:

7.2.1 knowledgeably discuss the advantages of the policies at St. Anthony's maternity unit

8.0 Objective

By the end of this class, the couple will rehearse strategies for labor.

8.1 Teaching Strategies

The instructor will:

8.1.1 create various labor situations that underscore key points in the preparation for childbirth series

8.1.2 direct these situational questions to the group for discussion

8.1.3 use appropriate visual materials such as birth atlas, knitted uterus, and labor graph to dispel any misconceptions couples may have

8.1.4 answer questions appropriately

8.2 Criteria

The client will:

8.2.1 participate in question and answer discussion led by instructor

8.2.2 answer correctly to appropriate situations

APPENDIX D

The following Recommendations were developed by working groups at the 1973 National Summer Working Conference of the American Society of Childbirth Educators held in Philadelphia Pennsylvania.

Task Group I: Guidelines for Labor Room Nurses Working With Prepared Couples

Task Group II: Guidelines for Physicians Working With Prepared Couples

Task Group III: Establishing Preparation for Childbirth Classes.

Task Group I
Guidelines for Labor Room Nurses Working with Prepared Couples

GROUP LEADER
GLADYS LIPKIN, RN, MS

I. INTRODUCTORY STATEMENT

Individualized care for the parent is an essential responsibility of the health team, which includes the childbirth educator, nurse, physician, as well as the mother herself. To implement this, it is essential that there be a sharing of information about the patient by all the members of the team. Consideration must be given to what the patient wants—her goals for this pregnancy—as well as her needs as seen by the team. The social, economic, cultural, health, and emotional factors of her environment should be included in the planning of her care.

II. NURSING TASKS THAT ARE MODIFIED WHEN THE PATIENT IS AWAKE

Members of the health team should modify some aspects of care in accordance with the goals of the mother. Whenever possible, her desire to be

306

medicated or not medicated, conscious or unconscious, prepared or not prepared in advance for childbirth, should be respected. Her need for the presence of a supportive person should be recognized and met. That person should be of her choice, whether husband, extended family member, nurse, childbirth educator, or friend, and should be accepted nonjudgmentally by the health team.

III. NURSING RESPONSIBILITIES THAT ARE NOT MODIFIED WHEN THE PATIENT IS AWAKE

The professional health team has to be accountable for the identification of clues to physiological and emotional processes that will affect the health and well-being of mother and baby. The professionals cannot abrogate responsibility for watching and measuring the processes. Tasks include checking the fetal heart rate, maternal blood pressure, pulse, etc., whether with standard tools such as the stethoscope or sophisticated equipment such as the fetal monitor. All members of the team should work as a consortium for the health and well-being of the mother and child, to provide a safe and dignified labor and delivery. Reporting and recording information is essential to this sharing.

Comfort measures for the patient in the labor room are not modified by her state of wakefulness, nor the presence of a supportive person. The patient may need reinforcement of her previously learned techniques or may need instant teaching of techniques. In either case, the health team member must be able to teach and demonstrate the material clearly and effectively.

If a nonprofessional supportive person is present in the labor room, his needs for support must be considered. Frequently communication with the patient must be channeled through this individual to be received correctly by the patient. This is particularly true when the supportive person has been prepared for childbirth with the patient.

Contact with other family members not present in the labor room should be maintained by a health team member. They, as well as the patient, should be kept aware of her progress.

If the patient has been prepared for the childbirth experience it is likely that she will have less need for anesthesia or analgesia. Any information about the extent of her training should be shared by the team members. This sharing cannot be modified, regardless of the state of the patient.

IV. WAYS TO FACILITATE EXTRAMURAL COMMUNICATION

There should be a collaborative effort between childbirth educators and hospital staffs to share their approaches and methods of instruction and care. If the patient is considered to be the hub of the care, and all members of the team and other supportive persons as the spokes, all will make a concerted effort to work together with the patient. No team member should undermine the work of another—nor would any one want to, if the patient's safety and welfare is the focus. Whenever possible, the childbirth educator should be offered the chance to visit hospital or home facilities used for labor and delivery by her patients. Similarly, in order to integrate all the supportive team members, the hospital members should be offered the chance to visit, and perhaps teach, childbirth classes.

It would be helpful for contacts to be set up between members of the health team, as well as between those members and the patient, along with any supportive person chosen by the patient. This would then focus on the needs and expectations of each of the persons involved, and could be used as a guideline for the planning of care.

V. RESOURCES FOR IMPROVING DIRECT PATIENT-CARE PRACTICES WITH ONGOING EVALUATION

The starting point for improving patient-care practices should begin early in life. Society should provide opportunities for human sexuality and family planning rather than with the identification of a pregnancy. The health team should be involved in the prenatal care, teaching whatever is necessary for patient care, and individualizing that care to assure the safety and comfort of the patient.

Any evaluation must consider the patient's perception of her care, for she will not accept that care unless it meets her needs as she sees them. Peer evaluation by professionals helps to reinforce positive aspects of care, and motivates the health team to upgrade their level of care. The patient's comments should receive top priority in bringing about effective change in her prenatal, perinatal, and postnatal care.

Task Group II
Guidelines for Physicians Working with Prepared Couples

GROUP LEADER
THOMAS J. VALIN, MD

I. INTRODUCTORY STATEMENT

By and large physicians practice their specialty in a manner very much the same as that practiced in the area of their training. Methods of practice are altered usually by the local environment in a new location or by changes in the doctors' philosophy towards the methods used in fulfilling their responsibilities in childbirth.

There seems to be little doubt in the great majority of practicing obstetricians that the pregnancy care process is a time-consuming event. Coupled with the many prenatal visits, extra consultations and postpartum visit, the delivery itself, which often arrives at an unopportune time, is an uncompromising event in the daily schedule of a busy obstetrician.

Obstetrician–gynecologists are in great demand today, especially in the rural and semiurban areas. Journals list many openings for the newly licensed specialist. The decreasing birthrate nationally coupled with the increasing abortion rate will not in any way simplify our objective of creating an interest and a desire in the practicing physician to accept the concepts of prepared childbirth as we understand them. Physicians are always pressed for time. If participation requires more of their time our aim must be to produce precise guidelines to present to them for their study and use.

309

The overall picture, at the present time at least, is an inadequate number of new specialists, poorly trained in the newer concepts of the psychoprophylactic method of childbirth, added to an overworked, and often uninterested, group of practicing obstetricians. If physicians are not trained during their mandatory educative years in trained childbirth methods, our outlook will be bleak indeed. The fulfilling experience of working with a trained couple during their younger training years, may be the one single event responsible for their full participation in later years.

Our direction of action is very clear: Education of the fledgling student and the practicing physician and most important, to modify the thinking of so many of the practicing physicians who look upon any trained childbirth method as a return to unrealistic individualism of days gone by.

II.   MEDICAL TASKS THAT ARE MODIFIED

A. Awareness of the overall concepts involved
   1. Participation (at least at the local level) in professional educator meetings or reading material made available by local educators
   2. Being available to act as medical advisor to professional teaching groups
   3. Accept childbirth education classes as an extension of offered routine practice courses
B. Changes in office management
   1. Very little to no change except for a compassion towards the couple who have chosen the psychoprophylactic method of delivery
   2. Simple signing of health clearance forms to attend approved childbirth education classes
   3. Completion of forms required by the physician, releasing him of any and all liability that may occur in this method of delivery, including the husband in the delivery room
   4. Dependence upon instructor groups to train adequately couples in the method used. Realization that many of the routine questions relative to the final trimester of pregnancy and labor onset will be answered by these instructors.
   5. Having available to new patients brochures that introduce them to the method and to the instructional team

6. Discussion relative to types of sedatives used in labor and choice of terminal anesthetics

C. Hospital management
1. Acceptance of the father as a member of the labor and delivery team:
   a. Labor
      i. Father's responsibilities are directed mainly towards the mother in caring for her needs and as a coach and constant observer
      ii. Husband is cognizant of his responsibility to nurse and physician and any hospital restrictions
      iii. Assurance that proper guidelines for hospital routines in order to maintain infection control have been established
      iv. Adjust sedatives to conform with ultimate aims of the prepared couple
   b. Delivery
      i. Father's presence, a physical and emotional support for mother; not as a viewer
      ii. Presence of the father not a detriment in difficult or complicated deliveries
      iii. Husband in the delivery room has not encouraged any legal actions; in fact, has enhanced a more cooperative effort between the physician and the family
      iv. Choice of technical anesthetic away from general towards local or regional block anesthetics
      v. Realization that the trained mother is better prepared to utilize practiced expulsive maneuvers to facilitate spontaneous delivery

III. MEDICAL RESPONSIBILITIES THAT ARE NOT MODIFIED

A. Office
1. Considering limited time and space, routine prenatal visits with the father are not essential except under certain circumstances
2. Office time schedule must be maintained. The prepared couple does not require additional office time
3. No changes recommended in the routine medical and laboratory work-up of the prenatal patient

B. Hospital
   1. Labor
      a. No demands made requiring additional labor visits, examinations, etc.
      b. Husband's presence not to deter from physician's routine schedule of labor visits
      c. Ultimate use of medications in labor remain the physician's responsibility
      d. Labor inducement, when recommended by the physician, for acceptable reasons, not a deterrent to the trained couple
   2. Delivery
      a. Physician delivery methods, including sterile techniques, draping, use of local or regional anesthetics need not be altered
      b. Physician management of obstetrical emergencies not altered with the prepared couple

IV. WAYS TO FACILITATE PROFESSIONAL COMMUNICATION

The physician interested in childbirth education must first have an understanding of the role of the professionals involved in the childbirth program. In this regard, he can be most beneficial and establish a direct line of communications by acting in an advisory capacity to the local childbirth educators and the involved hospital personnel. Through attending and participating in scheduled childbirth education classes, he can establish a better rapport with the above named team to fulfill best the needs of the prepared couple.

Further suggestions may include physician presentation to departmental staff meetings of nursing personnel or of physicians.

V. RESOURCES FOR IMPROVING PATIENT CARE

A. Evaluation of Patient Care
   1. Increased communication and involvement between labor and delivery nurses and childbirth educators

2. More data collection
   a. hard facts
   b. research studies
   c. longitudinal studies
3. Sensitizing institutional health professionals to changing parent needs
4. Parent feedback—parents to health professionals
   a. at the end of childbirth education class
   b. after labor and delivery
5. Evaluation of the parent feedback with the childbirth collaborative team.

Task Group III
Establishing Preparation for Childbirth Classes

GROUP LEADER
EDITH WONNELL, RN, CNM

INTRODUCTION: REASONING BEHIND TEACHING OR INTEREST IN CHILDBIRTH EDUCATION

I. PHILOSOPHY

A. Our initial aim is the education of the parents to the entire maturational cycle
B. Concern for the family and significant others as a unit
C. Maturation process of the family which is the recognition of individual parent's needs and helping them to achieve the goal they seek
D. The right to be well informed, which allows parents to make knowledge-able decisions concerning their health and that of their families as well

II.   CONSIDERATIONS FOR ESTABLISHING A PROGRAM

A. Assessment of the need
B. What is available in the community
C. Survey on the population (help administrator)
D. Central Unit—childbirth classes held in hospital
E. Receptability of the community
F. Understanding of socioeconomic group
G. Resource information and choosing instructors
H. Finances
I. Knowledge of policies
  1. physicians
  2. hospital

III.   WHO SHOULD TEACH, QUALIFICATIONS NEEDED

A. Group dynamics, art of communication
B. Previous pregnancy is not required
C. Knowledge of childbirth process
D. Practical experience in maternity nursing
E. Attitudes and interest, motivation important
F. Understanding of sociological aspects of childbirth
G. Knowledge of child growth and development
H. Philosophy of childbirth education

IV.   CONSIDERATIONS FOR ESTABLISHING POLICIES

A. Choosing class size may depend on the feeling of comfort the instructor has

B. Try to ventilate the feelings of the parents
   1. help class assistant (share her experience)
   2. male instructor (talk to the husbands)
   3. breaking down of the classroom type barrier
C. Length of class—6–8 weeks
   1. academic 1 hour/week
   2. practical 1 hour/week (6 hours/series minimum)
D. Fee schedules
   1. nonprofit service (adequate to cover cost)
   2. standard (one set fee)
E. Independent practitioner vs. employee
   1. Advantages to employee (consumer group) based classes
      a. administrative duties are relieved
      b. advisory board responsible for the quality of education
      c. resources
      d. prepared information
   2. Advantages of independent educator based classes
      a. expediency
   3. Advantages of institution (maternity hospital)
      a. continuity
      b. tours and parent familiarity with hospital
      c. use of resource people
      d. better feedback from staff and patients
      e. professional status
      f. better communication within hospital
      g. inservice workshop with nurses

V. FACILITATE COMMUNICATIONS BETWEEN PROFESSIONALS (CHILDBIRTH EDUCATION AND HOSPITAL PERSONNEL)

A. Hospital—emphasize team approach to care
B. Orientation program for all hospital personnel (obstetrician, nurses, nurses' aids, clerks, etc.)

C. Offer workshops for all nurses on breathing, coaching, and support techniques
D. Take advantage of opportunities to work on labor and delivery
   1. go in with patients
   2. work part-time in labor and delivery
   3. use labor room nurses as a possible pool of instructors or class assistants
E. Encourage patients to vocalize positive experiences to MD, nurses, administrators, etc. Encourage couples to write letters stating why they have changed hospitals or doctors.
F. Encourage formation of policy committees to set standards and review problems (MD, administration, RN, childbirth educators, etc.)
G. Encourage informal meetings/discussions between consumer group and professional group
H. Staff—evaluate couples' performance in labor and delivery
I. Have patients evaluate their own labor experience

Index

319